A COMPL**e** **g**UIDE FOR
FIRST-TIME MOMMIES

A COMPLETE GUIDE FOR FIRST-TIME MOMMIES

Healthy Pregnancy, Hospital Preparation, Post-Delivery Care

ANNE MARCELINE YEPMO

iUniverse, Inc.
Bloomington

A Complete Guide For First-Time Mommies
Healthy Pregnancy, Hospital Preparation, Post-Delivery Care

iUniverse books may be ordered through booksellers or by contacting:

iUniverse
1663 Liberty Drive
Bloomington, IN 47403
www.iuniverse.com
1-800-Authors (1-800-288-4677)

ISBN: 978-1-4620-7104-3 (sc)
ISBN: 978-1-4620-7106-7 (hc)
ISBN: 978-1-4620-7105-0 (ebk)

Printed in the United States of America

iUniverse rev. date: 12/15/2011

CONTENTS

INTRODUCTION

As a parent, your responsibility starts several months before your newborn baby arrives home from the hospital. During the nine months of your pregnancy, you are responsible for eating properly so as to provide proper nutrients for your growing, developing baby. You will need to take prenatal vitamins and keep away from some foods that might be harmful if eaten during pregnancy. Don't worry, the nine months will pass quickly and it will be great pleasure knowing you are doing everything possible to make your baby happy!

During your pregnancy, you should keep all of your doctor-appointments and make sure you follow your doctor's advice and guidance. This way, you will learn a lot about your baby's development during the nine months that you carry him/her in your womb. Wouldn't you want to learn the developmental stages of your newborn? This guide will help answer the questions you have about what is normal and what is not during pregnancy and post-delivery stages. It will help you understand what goes on in your body during pregnancy and provide you with tips for a healthy and happy pregnancy.

You do everything possible to keep your unborn baby safe, healthy and provide the backdrop for a healthy and happy life. Nothing seems like too much of a sacrifice for the safety and well-being of your precious little one. But sometimes you will have questions that haven not occurred to you before. This guide will help answer those questions and assure you that what you are experiencing is normal and healthy.

The day you bring your baby home from the hospital, is a very exciting and happy day. It is the beginning of your new life, as a parent, bringing up your child. But it is not uncommon for a new mom to be a bit worried on that day. In hospital, you and your new born were always surrounded by nurses and doctors. You could ask questions and the hospital staff would have all the answers. You may wonder what you will do if something "goes wrong" once you get home. You may worry that perhaps you will forget to take right precautions, fail to make right decisions, or accidentally hurt your baby by doing something wrong. You may feel you are not well prepared and do not know exactly what you should expect. Rest assured that it is not unusual for new moms to feel this way. Feelings of uncertainty do not mean you are not a good mom. Even your own mom probably felt somewhat insecure when she brought you home from the hospital.

Once you arrive home, you would want to enjoy and cherish every moment with your new baby. It will be a lifestyle adjustment, but it is important to remember that taking care of a baby comes very naturally to the new mommy. Earlier preparations and common sense go a long way toward caring for a baby. Babies have very simple needs and you will quickly master the art of meeting those needs. As your baby's needs change, you will adapt and learn how to care for the baby during that particular developmental stage of his/her life. Life is never dull once you become a mommy! This guide will be a constant companion and reference to help and guide you as a news mom.

When you arrive home from hospital, you would want to be relaxed as much as possible so your baby does not feel your tension or uncertainty. The best thing to do, before bringing your baby home from the hospital, is to make sure that you are fully prepared for this new "guest" in your home. Advance preparation will help alleviate a lot of anxiety and doubt; it will also make you confident that you are indeed ready and able to take good care of your baby.

Reading this guide is a great way to prepare yourself physically and mentally for child-birth and build your confidence. The guide will answer all of your new-mom questions and give you step-by-step instructions that are easy to read, memorize, and follow. The guide will also serve as an excellent reference when you need to quickly look up some information on taking care of your baby. This guide will go a long way in relieving your anxiety and helping you enjoy your baby-time.

Congratulations on taking steps to prepare for being the best mommy!

1

A HEALTHY, HAPPY PREGNANCY

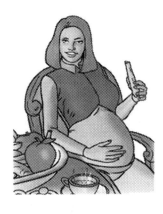

Your Pregnancy is Unique

It takes a while to get used to the idea that you are actually pregnant. If this is your first pregnancy, then you will be faced with many unfamiliar changes and uncertainties. It can seem unreal that there is actually another human being growing within you. If you have talked to other women about their pregnancy experiences, you have probably heard some women say; their pregnancy was a happy and fun nine months that they truly enjoyed. And you have probably heard others say that they were miserable throughout their pregnancy and it seemed to drag on and on for them. Every woman is different and so are their pregnancies. It is definitely not fair to develop negative, preconceived ideas about pregnancy based on others' experiences. Your experience will be your own. If your mother and other relatives have told you that they had an unhappy pregnancy and that it runs in the family, do not think that it means you will inevitably have an unhappy or difficult pregnancy too. While you do not have control over some things, in part, your pregnancy is what you make it. If you develop a good attitude right from the start, and ignore the negative things you hear about pregnancy, you will fare much better compared to deciding it is going to be a negative experience even before you go through it.

Part of the misery that some women experience may stem from the fact that during the first pregnancy, they may not understand all pregnancy-related changes that happen in their body. Being informed can help alleviate fears and anxiety over the changes that are happening, and put you at ease. As previously stated, there are some things that you do not have any control over, but there are many things that you can do to stay safe, healthy, comfortable and happy during the pre-delivery months.

Remember; every woman is different. Your body type is different. Your baby is different. Your lifestyle is different. Same things do not work for everyone. If one thing does not work to help you stay comfortable and happy, try something different. This chapter is loaded with great tried and tested tips to help make your first pregnancy a breeze. One that you will always remember with fondness.

Healthy, Happy Pregnancy Tips

♦ **Start with a Positive Attitude**
Your attitude at the beginning of your pregnancy can greatly affect how your pregnancy period goes. Your attitude during pregnancy also affects your baby. Studies show that women who are stressed during pregnancy are at higher risk of giving birth to low-weight babies. According to a June 2008 news release by ANI, Professor Vivette Glover; the lead researcher behind an exhibit from the Institute of Reproductive and Developmental Biology at Imperial College in London, says a mother's stress and anxiety can affect the development of an unborn baby's brain, therefore resulting in higher risk of emotional and behavioral problems. Your positive attitude certainly makes a huge difference and can help your little one start their life on a positive note!

Try to develop a positive mindset that pregnancy is not only about gaining weight, morning sickness, and moodiness. While these things can be a part of pregnancy, there are also many happy things to focus on. Focus on the fact that there is a precious, tiny baby growing and developing within you. Your pregnancy is a time of bonding with your baby, getting to know your baby. Sing happy songs to your unborn baby. Touch your tummy and talk to your baby. While in the womb, your baby may learn to recognize your voice.

Accept your pregnancy, your baby and your new role as a mother. Tell your baby that you love them and are happy to be their mommy. Express feelings that let your baby know that you welcome and cherish him/her. Your baby doe not understand words yet, but he/she understands emotions. He/she can understand what you are feeling toward him/her.

If you are having a difficult time accepting your baby or your role as a mother, talk to a counselor or your doctor. Be honest about how you feel. There is nothing "bad" about the feelings you have. Maternal feelings may not instantly develop. With all the hormonal upheaval that happens during the first trimester of pregnancy, you may need some help in sorting out your feelings. Counselors understand this and can help you come to reasonable conclusions and solutions.

Some women, especially those who did not plan their pregnancy, say they feel their lives and bodies are suddenly being taken over by their unborn baby. They feel deprived of being their own person and having lost possession and control of their own body. Some feel, they have suddenly become the hostess for another living creature, while they themselves fade into the background. Some others feel overwhelmed with the responsibility for the well-being, health and safety of another human being. If you experience these feelings, do not stuff them deep down inside or ignore them. Talk to a counselor about your feelings. This will help avoid feelings of resentment and be best for you and your baby.

It is estimated that approximately half of all pregnancies are unplanned. Whether planned or not, once you are pregnant, you cannot turn back the clock; but you can certainly make the best of your pregnancy! Instead of dreading or fearing it, or imagining negative things based on other's stories, rejoice in the process of creation, in wonders of nature that has given you this power of creation! Think positive, have a positive imagination and speak positive things about your baby and your delivery.

Enjoy your pregnancy. It may help considerably if you seek out and get together with other first-time moms. You can meet other expectant moms at childbirth classes, at doctor's appointments, and church groups. Ask around about new-moms groups. You may even want to start one in your neighborhood with other first-time moms.

- **Develop a support team.** Do not go through your pregnancy alone. Of all the times in your life when you will need an occasional shoulder to cry on, need someone to share exciting moments with, need occasional help and support—it is most needed during your pregnancy. Even if you have a terrific significant other who is supportive and helpful, develop some outside help and support-people also. This will give your partner a break and also provide you with fresh perspectives and ideas when you need them.
- **Tame morning sickness.** Sure, it is called *morning* sickness, but it can actually occur at any time of the day or night and it may be the most complained about issue of pregnancy. Although morning sickness can occur at various levels and some women do not experience morning sickness at all, most pregnant women experience it to some degree.

As the name implies, morning sickness seems to be most prevalent in the mornings upon waking up. If you are experiencing morning sickness, prepare for it the night before by putting a trash bag-lined wastebasket next to your bed. If eating saltines or ginger crackers and drinking ginger ale helps, you should also keep them on your bedside table the night before.

Usually morning sickness is most prevalent during the first trimester of pregnancy, but some women may experience it throughout their pregnancy. Sometimes it goes away for a period and then comes back. Its intensity also differs. Some women experience a nauseated feeling, much like the feeling one gets when they have motion sickness. Others throw up. Morning sickness does not hurt your baby, but you need to make sure you stay hydrated if you are vomiting. If you are losing a considerable amount of weight or if the vomiting becomes severe, be sure you consult with your doctor. With morning sickness, the phrase, "this, too, shall pass" will help you remember that the condition is temporary!

Remedies for Morning Sickness

If you are not among those fortunate ones who escape morning sickness, there are many remedies to provide you some relief:

- o Avoid greasy or spicy food or other foods that make you feel sick.

o Eat smaller meals about every two to three hours instead of larger meals.

o Do not drink anything while you are eating your meal. Drink plenty of water between meals.

o Do not skip meals. Keep high-protein snacks, such as cheese, with you at all times so you can have a snack whenever you start to feel hungry.

o Eat a few plain saltine crackers or ginger crackers before you get out of bed in the morning.

o Ginger can be beneficial in warding off nausea. Drink ginger tea or ginger ale, use ginger while cooking, eat baked goods which contain real ginger (not ginger flavoring). You can also purchase ginger capsules at health food stores.

o Avoid warm, stuffy rooms.

o Avoid smells that trigger nausea.

o Use citrus essential oil air sprays or sniff a handkerchief that has been sprayed with lemon or lime juice.

o Get out of bed slowly in the mornings, avoid any sudden movements.

o Avoid fast movements at any time of the day or night.

o Avoid fatigue and stress, which can increase the intensity of morning sickness.

♦ **Remember to have fun and enjoy your pregnancy.** Nine months are a long time to "hold your breath and wait for the pregnancy to be over." The time will pass much faster and you'll be much happier if you embrace your pregnancy and decide to enjoy it. Do not forget to have fun while you are pregnant. You are pregnant—not sick. Do not stop doing the positive activities that you did before you became pregnant; as long as they are safe for you and the baby. Continue to go out and meet with positive friends, work, exercise, play, dabble in hobbies. Do not lose your individuality in the excitement over your baby. Rather than put your life on hold during pregnancy, incorporate pregnancy into your life.

♦ **Maintain your standard of personal hygiene and beauty.** Pregnant women have a natural glow about them that makes them truly beautiful. Many women are happy to find that their prenatal vitamins improve their hair and skin. And yet, pregnant women often complain that they feel so fat and ugly during pregnancy. To help avoid this feeling, buy attractive, comfortable maternity clothes that you are happy to wear. The clothes do not need to be expensive, especially if you do not intend to wear them through a second pregnancy. But comfort is important. And fortunately, designers now create comfortable yet stylish maternity clothes that are suitable for casual or business wear.

Do not be tempted to get sloppy with your appearance or personal hygiene just because you may not have as much energy as you did before. Take time to look your best so that you will feel your best.
Do not isolate yourself or turn down social invitations just because you do not want to get dressed up. You'll feel better about yourself and about being pregnant if you pay attention to your appearance and continue to live your social life as you did before pregnancy, as long as you are still getting plenty of rest and sleep.

- ♦ **Do not obsess over weight-gain.** Do not get upset over the fact that you will gain weight during your pregnancy. It is absolutely natural and necessary for you to gain some weight during your pregnancy. Your body has to gain weight in order to provide what nourishment baby needs and keep him/her safe. Remember, your baby is constantly growing! You also need to store up some extra fat for delivery and breastfeeding your baby.

It is true that you are eating for two, so do not stress if, within reason, you want to eat more often and larger portions than you did before. Eat plenty of healthy, nourishment-rich foods and stay away from sugary, high-calorie foods and junk food. Do not panic over the pounds gained. If you feel you are gaining too much weight, talk to your doctor about it. You may need to change what you are eating.

On an average, women gain between 25-35 pounds during pregnancy. Usually, the baby accounts for about seven to eight pounds of the weight. Now do not panic—rest of the weight is not all fat accumulating in your stomach area and on your hips! The amniotic fluid can weigh around two pounds; the placenta weighs about one-and-one-half pounds, the uterus weighs about two pounds, as does breast tissue. There is an increase in blood volume that contributes about four pounds to the weight gain, and about seven pounds is gained because of storage of fat, protein and nutrients needed for delivery and breastfeeding. Even if you do gain a few extra pounds over the 25-35 pounds, you will be able to lose the extra weight after the baby is born. (Faster weight loss after the delivery is another advantage of breast feeding your baby).

♦ **Deal with moodiness.** Your body becomes a bundle of busy hormones when you are pregnant. This can create mood swings. You may find yourself acting like someone you do not know! And your partner will probably give you a few "what is going on" looks during your pregnancy. One minute you may be laughing and the next minute you may burst into tears. It helps to understand that this is quite normal and you are not going insane! Let your partner know that moodiness is a normal part of pregnancy and that you'll do what you can to control your moodiness; but also, that you would appreciate an extra measure of understanding and patience.

There are some things you can do to reduce extreme moodiness while you are pregnant:

o **Get plenty of rest and sleep.** When you are tired, it is more difficult to deal with the hormonal fluctuations and you may become tense, irritable and unable to cope with outbursts. During your pregnancy you will need more sleep and rest than you normally do so as to keep away a sleep deficit. Adjust your amount of sleep so you can feel well rested. Try to take twenty-minute naps during the day or after work. You may want to start going to bed an hour earlier or sleeping an hour more in the mornings. Getting enough sleep is absolutely critical while you are pregnant.

Learn to take mini breaks. If you are out shopping, find a chair or bench and rest while you sip on some water and have a healthy snack. Ask your partner to rub your shoulders or your feet for a few minutes after work or after you have been on your feet cooking or cleaning house. Mini massages can help increase blood flow and energize your body. Take warm baths (not too hot) and relax for ten to twenty minutes whenever you can. Sip on hot herbal tea while you are working. It will help relaxing your body. Even just resting your head on your desk for ten minutes during your lunch break can go a long way toward restoring your energy for the afternoon.

Avoid using caffeine-drinks for energy bursts just to keep going when you are tired and sleepy. If you feel tired and sleepy—take rest or sleep. Caffeine-drinks can wreak havoc with your hormones and affect your sleep at night. Caffeine may give you a burst of energy, but once the caffeine buzz wears off, you'll crash hard.

- o **Eat a healthy diet.** Not only a healthy diet will help keep weight-gain in check, it will also help keep your blood sugar levels stable. Eat fresh fruit and lots of vegetables of various colors, lean meat and other forms of protein such as eggs and peanut butter, high-fiber whole grains such as oats and bran, legumes, and dairy products such as yogurt and milk.

A poor diet, that makes blood sugar levels rise and fall, can contribute to moodiness, irritability, confusion fogginess and inability to cope well with everyday tasks and issues. That is the last thing you want.

  - o So avoid sodas and other sugary drinks such as juice-drinks that contain high fructose corn syrup and little or no real fruit.
  - o Avoid indulging in simple carbohydrates such as cake, candy, doughnuts and pie very often. If you do eat an occasional treat, eat half portions.
  - o For healthier eating, replace white pasta with whole grain pasta; replace some white potatoes with nutrient-packed yams; replace white bread with whole grain bread; replace sugary drinks with herbal tea or water.

A Tuft University study also found that not drinking enough water can have a negative effect on your mood. True, drinking more water will mean more trips to the bathroom, and that does get tiresome when you are pregnant. But do not avoid drinking water, even when you are away from home just because of the bathroom issue. Drinking plenty of water is necessary for over-all good health. Plus, if you are breastfeeding your baby, you will need to be in the habit of drinking a lot of water and liquids. If you have clean, pure tap water, it is fine to continue drinking tap water. If you travel or go any place where you are uncertain about the water, it is best to drink bottled water.

The best way to develop a habit of drinking enough water is to stop drinking anything but water. Sometimes, when you are accustomed to reaching for a soda or other drinks, you do not realize how little water you actually drink.

o **Pace yourself.** If your schedule is so hectic that you never have time for yourself or time to relax, you may start feeling overwhelmed. Slow things down while you are pregnant. Try not to pack more into a day than you can manage without feeling stressed or unbalanced. Staying balanced is the key—you do not want to stop everything, but you do not want to be too busy, either.

If you are not up to certain tasks while you are pregnant, do not be afraid to admit it and make changes and alternative plans. For example, Cathy's parents were having their 50th wedding anniversary when she was seven months pregnant. Cathy was a professional caterer, so she always prepared food for all family events. Cathy's siblings assumed she would cook for the wedding anniversary too. Cathy wanted to prepare food for a special banquet for her parents' anniversary. But she knew, in order to prepare food for over 100 people, it would require her to be on her feet for three or four days before the event, not to forget servicing her other clients as well. Instead of not participating at all, Cathy thought of an alternate plan that she felt she could comfortably manage. She told her siblings that she could not manage a full banquet, but with their help she could manage a formal dessert celebration.

Avoid emotionally-charged or difficult situations whenever you can. Try not to take on other people's problems. Prioritize so that you take care of the really important things, and let the other things go.

Remember to always breathe deeply and exhale slowly to keep your body oxygenated, and try to keep everything in perspective, especially on more challenging days.

○ **Talk to someone about your feelings, ask your questions.** If you feel overwhelmed, call your mother, your sister, a good friend, or a trusted co-worker and talk to them about how you are feeling. It is okay to cry on someone's shoulder once in a while. You'll always feel better after a good cry that allows you to release pent up emotions.

○ Do not be embarrassed to ask questions of other moms or your doctor. No question is too insignificant. Of course you can do research online, but you cannot always find the specific answer you are looking for. If you do online research, be aware that anyone can put information on a website, whether it is accurate or true information or not. Make sure you check only reliable medical and pregnancy information sites.

○ **Exercise.** Exercise is beneficial for pregnant women on many levels. In addition to helping you stay in shape throughout your pregnancy, which in turn, will make your delivery easier, the body releases endorphins when you exercise and endorphins improve your mood.

 The American College of OB-GYN states that some amount of exercise is safe during pregnancy. However, during pregnancy you should not do exercises which restricts blood flow and require you to lie on your back, as this can cause the uterus to contract. The danger in that is if the contractions continue then it can induce pre-mature labor pain.

When you exercise, it is important to stay hydrated. If you are not used to exercising, start with a gentle exercise program, not a rigorous one. Walking, recreational swimming, gentle yoga and gentle water aerobics provide excellent exercise for pregnant women. Even though it may seem like a lot of trouble to take the time for exercise every day, the benefits far outweigh the trouble!

o **Pray, Meditate, Sing**, or do whatever you do for spiritual well being. Take a time out. Light a candle and take a warm bath. Go sit in your favorite place all by yourself. Allow yourself the time to do something special, such as sit and read a book without interruptions or take a walk. Take the time to do whatever you do to help restore peace and sanity.

♦ **Avoid becoming sick.** During your pregnancy, do whatever you can to avoid coming down with a cold, flu or other common sickness. Take precautions and wash hands frequently. Keep your immune system built up by eating a healthy diet, drinking lots of water, and taking your prenatal vitamins. Avoid contact with people who are sick. If you work in a public environment where you are constantly exposed to people who are sick, take extra precautions.

During your pregnancy avoid exposure to chemicals, including household chemicals, and environmental toxins such as cigarette smoke and paint fumes. If you do gardening, always wear protective gloves while working with soil, avoid gardening chemicals such as insecticides. Same goes for any strong chemical you would use for hobbies.

♦ **Do not smoke, drink, or use drugs.** Make an immediate and firm decision that your baby's health comes first and stop all smoking, drugs and alcohol during your pregnancy. Cigarettes, drugs, and alcohol in your system can severely harm your baby and cause low birth weight and complications that lead to long-term problems or even death. This goes for second-hand smoke also, so steer clear of other smokers and smoky environments.

If you are taking prescription medication, tell your doctor about the meds as soon as you find out that you are pregnant. If your doctor says that your medication is safe for you to take during pregnancy, make sure you follow your doctor's instruction to the letter. Avoid taking any over-the-counter drugs unless your doctor has specified that the drug is permissible during your pregnancy.

If you need more information on how smoking, drugs, and alcohol use can affect your unborn baby, ask your doctor for literature on the topic, or do your own online research. If you are addicted to any drugs, make sure you talk to your doctor about it and for recommendations on how you can come clean. Your baby's life is at risk if you continue to use drugs during your pregnancy.

♦ **Avoid x-rays.** This includes dental x-rays. If it is absolutely necessary for you to have x-rays, make sure the dentist knows that you are pregnant and takes every possible precaution for minimal exposure and safety.

♦ **Avoid stress.** Everyone experiences some stress in their lives, but during your pregnancy you should try to avoid stress as much as possible. Do not make choices and decisions that will lead to stress. Be quick to find solutions and remove yourself from stressful circumstances when you can. Do not hesitate to say 'no' about situations that you know will be stressful for you. For example, if you have a younger sister who wants to come and stay with you during summer vacation, but you know she is having some behavioral problems which would be stressful for you, say no or suggest an alternate plan. An alternative might be for your sister to spend a few weekends or one week with you instead of the whole summer.

Right from the start of your pregnancy, determine that your health and the health of your baby are going to be your main priority. Others may not understand this decision, but that is not your problem. Your pregnancy is not the time for you to take on others' problems.

♦ **Do not take very hot baths or go in a hot tub or sauna.** It is okay to take warm baths, but your bath-water should not be over 100 degrees Fahrenheit. As a general rule of thumb, your foot should feel comfortable when you put it in the bath-water. If your foot stings from the hot water, it is too hot. According to Jeanne-Marie Guise, an OB-GYN, if the bath water is too hot, it will cause an increase in your heart rate, reduce blood flow to the fetus and potentially put the baby under stress. Hot tubs and saunas are too hot and completely off-limits during pregnancy.

♦ **Use safe hygiene practices.** Avoid scented feminine hygiene products. Use natural unscented sprays, sanitary napkins, powders, soaps and bath products to avoid irritating the vaginal area and increasing risk of a urinary tract infection or yeast infection.

Do not douche during your pregnancy as it can irritate the vagina and create risk of infection. Keep the vaginal area dry (free from moisture) and clean. Wear looser cotton-crotch panties to further cut down on risk of infections.

♦ **Do not attempt to clean a cat litter box or rodent cage.** If you try to clean out a cat litter box, you are risking toxoplasmosis, which is an infection that can be harmful to your unborn baby. If you do gardening or have any other reason to dig in the dirt, wear protective gloves and thoroughly wash your hands afterward.

Rodents such as mice, hamsters and guinea pigs can carry a virus that is very harmful or even deadly to your unborn baby. Do not clean out rodent cages or allow yourself to come in contact with any area which might have rodent droppings or urine.

♦ **Communicate with medical professionals; keep all your prenatal appointments.** As soon as you suspect that you are pregnant or have taken a home pregnancy test or other pregnancy test that confirms that you are pregnant; set an appointment to see a doctor or midwife for prenatal (pregnancy) care. Women who receive prenatal care have much better chance of delivering a healthy, full-term baby, as opposed to women who wait till late in their pregnancy to receive care, or do not receive care until delivery.

　o **What happens in prenatal visit?**

　　- On your first prenatal visit, your health care professional will do a complete physical exam that includes a pelvic exam.

You will also be asked to complete paperwork that includes questions about your health history and your family's health history. You will be asked to provide a urine and blood sample which will be sent to a lab. The exciting part of your first visit is that the doctor will calculate your due date! You may still be having a hard time believing that you are actually pregnant, but having a due date will help your pregnancy seem more real to you. It will also allow you to plan ahead.

- Also, on your first prenatal visit, your doctor will give you a prescription for prenatal vitamins or tell you what vitamins to use. Make sure you follow through by getting and taking the prenatal vitamins right away. It is important to note that whatever prenatal vitamins your doctor prescribes or recommends should contain 400 mcg of folic acid. Studies show that folic acid may prevent birth defects that can happen during the first few months of pregnancy.

Sometimes first-time moms can have a difficult time communicating with their doctor. After all, you have never been pregnant before and you may not know exactly what you want to ask or say. That's ok. Just explain what you are feeling or ask questions in the simplest, day-to-day language. Knowing the terminology is their job! Do not be shy about asking questions or requesting more information.

Make a habit of writing down your questions as they come to your mind. Take your list to your next prenatal check up. Do not hesitate or be afraid that your questions are silly. This is a new experience for you. Your doctor is an ally and available to help you with any questions you might have.

It is extremely important for you and your baby's health and well-being that you keep all your prenatal appointments. You will be at peace when your doctor tells you all is going well. And if something does need attention, it is best that your doctor comes to know it as soon as possible. Your prenatal visits will usually be scheduled for once a month for the first seven months of your pregnancy. For the seventh and eighth months your doctor will probably schedule you for two visits per month, and during your ninth month and until birth, you will probably see your doctor weekly.

♦ **Keep a journal.** Writing about how you feel throughout your pregnancy can be therapeutic and help you keep things in perspective. The journal will also serve you in later years, to bring back the memories and details of your first pregnancy. The journal writing does not have to be a chore, and you don't have to fill any certain amount of pages per day or per week. It does not matter if you are good at writing or not, or if you flunked English classes in high school or college. The important thing is to get your feelings down on paper. Also, be sure to have plenty of your pictures are taken while you are pregnant. After all, it is the first time that you are pregnant and it will be wonderful to have its memories that you can cherish later!

Foods to Avoid During Pregnancy

You know what foods you should eat to stay healthy and help your baby grow and develop, but during your pregnancy there are also some foods that you should avoid:

➢ **Unwashed fruit or vegetables** should not be eaten as the soil they are grown in could contain toxoplasmosis. Always wash vegetables and fruit thoroughly before eating.

➢ **Deli meats** can be contaminated with bacteria called listeria. Listeria can enter the placenta and may infect the baby and possibly result in miscarriage.

➢ **Unpasteurized milk** can also contain listeria. Drink only pasteurized milk and juices.

➢ **Soft cheeses** are also known to sometimes contain listeria. Avoid cheeses such as feta, gorgonzola, brie, camembert, and Roquefort. Also avoid Mexican cheeses such as queso blanco, unless they are made from pasteurized milk.

➢ **Raw shellfish**, such as clams, oysters and mussels are often undercooked and cause problems. Even properly cooked shellfish should be avoided.

➢ **Raw meat or undercooked meat** can contain e-coli and other bacteria that can be harmful to your baby. Cooking meat at high temperatures usually destroys the harmful bacteria.

> ➤ **Raw eggs or foods that contain raw eggs** should not be eaten because of the risk of salmonella. Mayonnaise, custards, and Hollandaise sauce are common foods that are made with raw eggs.
> ➤ **Fish with high mercury levels** including swordfish, king mackerel, shark and tilefish should not be eaten. Canned tuna is controversial, but is believed to be safe if eaten in moderation during pregnancy.
> ➤ **Caffeine** amounts should be closely monitored or completely avoided. There have been some studies that show caffeine in large amounts may be related to miscarriages, low birth weight, and even withdrawal symptoms in newborns. Caffeine also eliminates fluid from the body, so you are risking dehydration if you drink too much caffeine.

Is it Safe to have Sex While I'm Pregnant?

This is a common question that most first time moms ask. And rightfully so—as sex during pregnancy is an important issue. You'll be happy to know that in most cases, as long as you or your partner does not have any sexually transmitted diseases, having sex during pregnancy is perfectly safe and does not present a problem. Having sex and orgasm does not harm your baby, who is protected in your uterus by the surrounding amniotic fluid. However, if your doctor has told you not to have sex during your pregnancy, you should follow their advice. Your doctor may give such an order if you have a history of premature labor or birth, or if you have placenta previa—which is a condition where part of the placenta covers the cervix.

Although at times sex during pregnancy can be a bit awkward, it should not be painful, and there should not be vaginal bleeding. If there is vaginal bleeding call your doctor immediately. If your water breaks, do not have sex after the water breaks. When you have an orgasm, your uterus will contract. This is normal, of course. But if the contractions are painful or continue into a regular pattern, call your doctor.

Often, women are tired and are experiencing so many hormonal changes in their body during the first trimester of pregnancy that they are not very interested in having sex. If this is the case, talk to your partner so they understand that you are not rejecting them. Be honest and keep communication open regarding sex throughout your pregnancy. Communicating will help avoid misunderstandings, fears, and hurt feelings. If you decide to continue to have sex throughout your pregnancy, talk about what positions work or do not work as your baby grows. Learn to laugh when clumsy things happen. Develop and discuss about other romantic ways to make your relationship more intimate when intercourse is not desired. But do not ignore the sex issue for nine months. Remember, you and your partner were a couple before the pregnancy, and you'll still be a couple after the pregnancy. It is important that you go through the pregnancy together and in harmony, and that includes the sex issue.

What to Wear During Pregnancy?

The key word for maternity clothes is *comfort!* Your body will be going through a lot of changes and you do not want to exacerbate the discomfort of those changes by uncomfortable clothes and shoes. Yes, you want to look stylish and dress appropriately for work and for other occasions, but you still want to be comfortable. This does not mean you have to resort to sweat pants and tennis shoes. You can find comfortable stylish maternity jeans, tops, dresses, and skirts. Belly bands can be worn over the top of your unbuttoned regular pants or jeans to hold them up and extend the waist band. You can even find comfortable, supportive bras and maternity panties that are feminine-looking and pretty. But do make sure that the bras you wear are supportive and fit properly. Cotton panties or cotton-crotch panties will help keep the vaginal area dry and cut down on risk of yeast infections. It is best to avoid tight-fitting pants during pregnancy, as they tend to trap in moisture that can cause infections.

If your budget is tight, keep in mind that some large box stores carry far less expensive maternity clothes than the ones found at maternity boutiques. You may have a friend or close relative who bought maternity clothes and wore them once and does not plan on wearing them again. Many women resell their maternity clothes after wearing them once and this means you may be able to find clean, nice maternity clothes at resell stores or garage sales for a fraction of the cost.

You may love high heels and be willing to sacrifice comfort for style, but during your pregnancy, comfort should be given priority over fashion. Choose shoes that are comfortable and offer ankle and arch support. During your pregnancy, your balance will be slightly off, so you would want to avoid high heels or clunky shoes that could contribute to tripping or falling. Instead, choose attractive low-heeled shoes. Your lower back, knees, and ankles will thank you!

Large, packed purses can be a heavy load for a body that is already carrying extra cargo. Switch to a smaller bag and one that distributes weight more evenly across your shoulders, rather than placing all of the weight in one spot. Beware of lifting and carrying heavy computer bags or back packs also.

Should I Work During My Pregnancy?

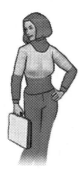

There was a time when women simply did not work once they found out that they were pregnant. But times have certainly changed and many women work up until their delivery time. Working during your pregnancy can help relieve any stress caused by loss of income, help you stay busy so that time passes quickly and most of all, keeps you physically active. Of course, whether you should work during your pregnancy and for how long, depends on your job and your individual health and situation. Discuss your job with your doctor and get their opinion on whether you should continue to work or not. Jobs that may not be suitable for pregnant women include:

> ➢ Jobs that require you to be exposed to infectious disease.
> ➢ Jobs that require you to be exposed to chemicals and toxic substances, including fumes or smoke.
> ➢ Jobs that require you to work in extreme weather or at extremely hot or cold temperatures.
> ➢ Jobs that are physically demanding and jobs that require climbing ladders, lifting heavy objects, or constant bending and stooping.
> ➢ Jobs that put you in a dangerous environment.
> ➢ Jobs that are extremely stressful.
> ➢ Jobs that require you to stand for more than three to four hours at a time.

Marcy loved her job as a kindergarten teacher. Every morning she looked forward to getting to class and greeting her young, energetic students. But after Marcy became pregnant, during the winter months, she was constantly sick with colds as her students often came to school with a cold. In order to keep working, Marcy had to take special precautions, which included asking her doctor how she could build up her immune system; practicing constant hand sanitizing; frequent sanitizing of classroom tools and supplies; as well as wearing a mask.

Most companies have set policies regarding pregnant employees. Read your employee handbook carefully and talk with your employer about special circumstances surrounding your job and your pregnancy. Explain that you may need to be excused for bouts with morning sickness and may need to take more frequent bathroom breaks. If your job requires that you wear a certain uniform, work out the maternity clothes details with your employer. Let your employer know that you will try to schedule doctor appointments outside of working hours, but may not always be able to do so. Comply with your company guidelines for putting in your request for maternity leave. Make sure your coworkers know when your due date is so they will understand how it will affect their jobs. Do whatever you can to make your work load lighter during the last few weeks of your pregnancy and have everything prepared in the event your baby decides to arrive early.

Sometimes adjustments can be made to make your job easier while you are pregnant. Even little changes, such as bringing in a footstool to raise your feet while working at your desk can make a difference. If company policy does not allow it otherwise, you may want to request permission to eat small snacks during the work day and to lie down in a comfortable place during your breaks.

If you find that working full time is too difficult or stressful during your pregnancy, talk to your employer about options such as working part time or doing part or all of your work from home. If your particular job is too strenuous, ask your employer to consider changing your position or job description for the duration of your pregnancy.

There are federal and state laws to help protect pregnant employees and to help them return to their job after having their baby. Check with your state employment division for state laws and also become familiar with the Pregnancy Discrimination Act, and the Family and Medical Leave Act.

According to the Pregnancy Discrimination Act, if your employer has 15 or more employees, they must provide the same rights for a pregnant woman as they provide for all other employees with medical conditions. This can be a two-edged sword because if your company does not provide benefits and security for other employees, it does not have to do so for you just because you are pregnant. The reason for this act is to make sure you are not treated *differently* just because you are pregnant. Under this act, you cannot be fired because you are pregnant, and you cannot be forced to take maternity leave if you choose not to. You must be given alternate assignments or modified tasks, disability leave, or leave without pay—whatever the company policy is. If you do take maternity leave, you are guaranteed job security during your leave, and during your leave you continue to remain eligible for benefits and pay raises and you continue to accrue seniority.

The Family and Medical Leave Act (FMLA) is applicable to companies with 50 or more employees. The act makes provision for up to twelve weeks of maternity leave with your job protected while you are away, any time during the first twelve-month period for the birth of your baby. There are many details surrounding the Family and Medical Leave Act. You can find the detailed information at the United States Department of Labor website at: http://www.dol.gov/whd/fmla/index.htm.

If you feel you are being discriminated against or treated poorly by other employees or superiors at your job because you are pregnant, you need to speak with your supervisor or company owner about it, as well as submit a formal written complaint. Deliver a copy of the complaint to the appropriate superiors, as well as e-mail it to them, and keep a copy for yourself. In this age and time, workplace discrimination against pregnant women may be rare, but it still does happen. Take necessary precautions to make sure you are protected in the event that the discrimination continues.

Understanding Your Pregnancy

You'll be much more relaxed if you understand all the new developments taking place in your body during each trimester of your pregnancy. By your doctor's calculations, from the start date of your last period, your pregnancy will be forty weeks. (That is a long time to wonder what's going on!) Forty weeks of pregnancy is divided into trimesters (three parts). There are distinct markers for each trimester.

First Trimester

This may sound really strange, but the way doctors calculate your due date, your baby hasn't actually been conceived during your first two weeks of pregnancy. Conception usually happens about two weeks after your period begins, and your period is counted as part of your pregnancy time. During the first twelve weeks, known as the first trimester, your body is changing and releasing hormones to get everything ready for your baby. You may experience some or all of these symptoms as a result of the hormonal changes:

- ✓ You will probably experience swollen, tender breasts and darkening around the nipples. This may be one of the first outward signs that you are pregnant.
- ✓ You will probably be fatigued—which may cause you to want to go to bed much earlier than you used to. You may actually think you are coming down with a cold or flu because you feel unusually tired.
- ✓ You may experience morning sickness, which includes an upset stomach and may include throwing up. Morning sickness does not just happen in the morning, but can happen at any time of day or night.
- ✓ You will probably experience moodiness to some degree, which may include feelings of wanting to laugh one minute and cry the next, or laughing or crying at inappropriate times. Even the most level-headed, organized person may start feeling a little out of control and overwhelmed.
- ✓ You may need to urinate more often than previously, with the feeling that you cannot wait very long once you need to urinate.

    ✓ There may be changes in what you like to eat or what smells you can tolerate. You may have cravings for certain foods that you may or may not have previously enjoyed, and want to eat them frequently. You may dislike foods or the smell of foods that you previously liked.

    ✓ You may experience headaches because of the hormonal changes.

    ✓ You may experience constipation.

    ✓ As your body makes necessary adjustments, you may experience weight loss or weight gain.

In case you have forgotten this from your Biology 101 class: during week three of your pregnancy, the sperm and egg come together and form a one-celled entity called a zygote. Your partner contributes 23 chromosomes to the zygote and you contribute 23. The chromosomes determine the gender of your baby as well as their hair and eye color. As the zygote travels down the fallopian tube, it divides and forms a cluster of cells. The inner cells of the cluster become the embryo and the outer cells become the protective and nourishing membranes. The zygote burrows itself into the uterine wall for nourishment, and the placenta starts to form. It is at this time, about the end of the fourth week, that your pregnancy test will show positive for pregnancy.

During the first trimester, your baby's spinal cord, brain, heart and other organs start to form, and your baby will be about the size of the tip of a pen by week five. The neural tube is closing and your baby's heart is pumping blood. Your baby's brain and face start to develop rapidly, and your baby's arms and legs are growing out from the tiny arm and leg buds, and fingers are forming. Your baby's eyes are also visible and the upper lip and nose have formed.

Your baby continues to grow and develop and by the ninth week, his/her arms develop bones, and tiny toes are beginning to form. By the tenth week, you may be able to hear your baby's heartbeat by ultrasound. Your baby's head is rounder and starts to look more like the big round head that is associated with babies. The neck also begins to develop. The baby's eyelids close to protect the eyes. Your baby's genitalia will start to develop.

As your first trimester ends, your baby will be around two-and-one-half inches long (from crown to bottom) and weigh about one-half an ounce.

Second Trimester

The second trimester consists of weeks 13 through 28. Many women tout the second trimester as the best part of their pregnancy. By that point, you have relaxed a little and feel like you have a grip on things. The baby has not grown to the point that you would feel huge and uncomfortable yet. There are some truly exciting moments during the second trimester. At around week 16, you will probably be able to tell your baby's gender from the ultrasound. At about 18 weeks, you will probably be able to feel your baby moving, even though your baby has actually been moving for some time. The movement may just feel like a flutter at first, but within a short time you will feel strong and definite movements. Your baby's movements will get more powerful as time goes on and you'll actually be able to feel when your baby is "kicking" or "punching."

✓ You may no longer be having morning sickness by this point.
✓ You may develop swollen ankles, fingers, and even your face may be a bit swollen.
✓ You may experience lower back pain and some pain in the thigh and groin.
✓ You may experience tingling in your hands and fingers.

Third Trimester

Once you are into your third trimester, weeks 29 through 40, you will probably start feeling excited about how close you are to the birth time. You may relax, feeling like you are on the home stretch, but things in your body will intensify again as you move into the latter part of the third trimester and your body prepares for the delivery.

✓ You may have a hard time getting comfortable due to the size of the baby. This may cause you to have problems sleeping. But it is important to stay as much rested as possible toward your due date. When you go to the hospital to deliver your baby, you'll need all the energy you can muster.

- ✓ You will probably need to go to the bathroom even more frequently as the baby begins to put pressure on your organs. You'll probably even plan around bathroom breaks, and know where every bathroom in town is at!
- ✓ You may also find that you experience shortness of breath because of the growing baby putting pressure on your organs. When walking, you'll probably stop fairly often to catch your breath.
- ✓ You may develop hemorrhoids. This is not uncommon. The hemorrhoids, which are swollen veins in and around the rectum, may even bleed at times. Since you have been warned that if there is any vaginal bleeding, any bleeding can be very scary during your pregnancy. It may be easy for you to discern that the bleeding is from the rectum. If you are not absolutely certain, call your doctor. Even if you are certain, let your doctor know that you have developed hemorrhoids.

  To help avoid hemorrhoids, drink plenty of water and eat high-fiber foods such as bran to keep bowel movements regular. To help relieve some of the discomfort of hemorrhoids, dip a cotton ball or pad in witch hazel and gently wipe the rectal area.

- ✓ Toward the end of your third trimester you may experience very tender breasts and the breasts may leak colostrums. Wearing disposable nursing pads will protect you from embarrassing surprises.
- ✓ You may notice that the baby is moving lower in order to get into position for birth. This is referred to as the baby dropping. You may feel like you are waddling when you walk, as the baby moves lower.

During the third trimester your baby will grow rapidly, going from about 1 ½ pounds at 25 weeks to about 71/2 or so pounds at birth. You'll find great comfort in knowing that your baby's lungs, brain and internal organs will mature to the point that he/she can survive on their own at 37 months.

2

IT'S ALMOST TIME!

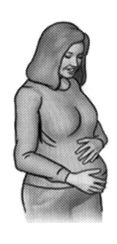

For the sake of brevity, let's assume that you are going to a hospital or birthing center to have your baby. If you are having a home birth, your preparation for birth and your birthing experience will be a bit different, though there will also be many similarities. Your midwife will give you clear instructions for preparing ahead of time for your home birth. Much of the information on preparing for birth and delivery is applicable whether you are going to the hospital or having a home birth. This guide will be beneficial either way. However, basic information about preparing for the hospital and your hospital stay is also provided in order to increase your confidence about the wonderful world of motherhood that you are about to enter.

Before you feel that magical moment and *know* that it is time to leave for the hospital, you'll want to be sure you have covered a few bases on the home front. Since first babies often do not come on their due date, unless you are having induced labor on a set date, you won't know exactly when you'll need to leave for the hospital. As you already know, babies may come a few days late or early, up to a couple of weeks late or early. This means you'll need to be as prepared as possible during your last month of pregnancy.

Personal Preparation

Since you have never had a baby before, it may be difficult for you to imagine all the things you should do before your baby is born. To some extent it depends on your personality. Are you the kind of person that is highly organized and wants everything done ahead of time? Are you the kind of person who likes to fly by the seat of her pants and see how things turn out? There are several lists and guidelines in this book; pick and choose what works for you and leave the rest. Adjust the lists to fit your personality, your lifestyle and your needs.

Some things to consider and take care of during your pregnancy:

➢ **Arrange maternity leave.** If you have a job or run your own business, make arrangements for maternity leave as much in advance as possible. If you run your own business, train someone to take your place for the amount of time you will need to be away or adjust your business to accommodate your absence. If you work for a company, make sure you understand the policy for maternity leave. You can usually find this information in your company handbook.

➢ **Make childcare arrangements if you work outside of the home.** If you will be returning to work after your baby is born, then you will need to seek out childcare arrangements. This can be a time-consuming process, so start the process early. It is a good idea to have a Plan B for childcare in case your first choice does not work out.

Some of your childcare choices may include public daycare centers, private in-home daycare center, or a family member or friend babysitting at your home or theirs. You may also opt to have a care provider come to your home while you work. In some instances, you and your partner may be able to work alternate shifts in order to avoid having someone else take care of your child. Even though many couples make that type of arrangement, it can take a toll on both parents, so do not make the choice lightly. Even if you choose to work in alternate shifts, you may want to have a back-up sitter for occasional relief to be able to spend time together.

Whatever you choose for child care; take every available precaution to ensure that your baby is left in safe, competent, caring hands. When you interview providers, ask specific questions. The answers given will help you know whether the person knows what they are talking about or not. Make sure the providers you consider have training specifically for infants and toddlers. Make sure to run a national criminal background check and thoroughly check all references provided by individual prospective child care providers. If you are hiring an in-home provider, as an added measure of safety consider having security cameras installed in your home. Many home and day care centers do have security cameras for their protection as well as your baby's. Video cameras allow parents to watch their baby in real time, online from their computers at work.

Whether your baby goes to day care or someone comes to your home, make unannounced visits at various times to see what is going on when you are not there. Make sure your child care provider does not smoke and that no one in the center or home smokes and exposes your baby to second hand smoke in the air or from their smoky clothes. Ask child care providers about first aid training, and once you have hired a provider, make sure they understand all emergency procedures.

➢ **Schedule appointments.** It may be important to you to look your best after the birth of your baby when you will have visitors at the hospital and after you get home. And you'll have very little time to go for a hair appointment after the baby is born. If you want to have your hair freshly cut and other beauty treatments, schedule appointments for a couple of weeks before your due date and you will probably be able to make the appointment. Be careful to follow all safety guidelines for beauty and spa appointments.

➢ **Arrange social calendar around due date.** If you have long-standing dates with friends or family, or once-a-year type meetings or events that will fall near your due date, let other participants know your due date and that, if you are missing at the date/event, it may be because you are at the hospital delivering your baby! Check your calendar for a few weeks past your due date and shop for birthday gifts and other special gifts and arrange for someone else to ship or deliver the gifts for you if needed.

➢ **Choose a name.** Unless you have made a conscious decision to not name the baby until after you have seen him/her, choose a name for your baby before you go to the hospital. At the hospital, you will need to put the baby's name on the birth certificate application form. If you choose names before you know the gender of the baby, choose both a boy's name and a girl's name. Do not forget to decide on the spelling of the name if it has multiple spellings.

➢ **Arrange for diaper service.** More moms are choosing cloth diapers again because they feel it is a sound, socially conscious decision to keep disposable diapers out of the landfill. In addition, more moms are concerned about the effect that the disposable diapers have on their infant's sensitive skin. If you are going to use a diaper service, arrange for the service several weeks before you leave for the hospital. Sometimes it can take a few weeks for a diaper service company to incorporate you into their delivery route.

Help Your Partner Prepare

Your pregnancy, delivery, hospital stay and coming home with an infant to care for will be much easier for your partner to cope with and help with if they also prepare before you go to the hospital. Given below is a list of things your partner can do:

✓ Give their employer notice of your due date and request time off from work during that time, or if they run their own business, train employees for their time away.
✓ Pack bag for hospital stay.
✓ With you, plan ahead financially.
✓ Attend doctor visits with you.
✓ Attend pregnancy classes with you.
✓ Do yoga or other pregnancy exercises with you.
✓ Read pregnancy books and discuss pregnancy and birth with you.

✓ If you are going to work after the baby is born, then help you interview and choose childcare provider.

✓ Memorize the stages of labor and know what will be going on in the delivery room.

✓ Know what his role will be in the delivery room.

✓ Help choose a name for your baby.

✓ Be informed about baby blues and postpartum depression so they can help you through it.

✓ Learn how to take care of newborns.

✓ Arrange for after-delivery help at home.

Nesting

Most mommies-to-be naturally start doing what is referred to as *nesting* during the last few weeks of their pregnancy. When moms nest, they have a desire to clean and organize everything at home. Even women who do not enjoy house cleaning may have a tendency to clean out closets and cupboards and organize like never before. They want everything to be clean and orderly for when the baby arrives! They want the nest to be prepared!

The nesting instinct is a good thing. Having things to do at home will help keep your mind and hands busy so you are not sitting around feeling anxious for the baby to arrive. Also, once you get home with your baby from the hospital, there will not be time for cleaning and organizing. You'll be very glad it is already done and you can enjoy adjusting to your new life with a baby.

 When you are cleaning and organizing during the nesting days before the delivery, be careful that you follow all safety rules. Do not use toxic or harsh cleansers or any substance with a very strong smell, even if it is a natural cleanser. Do not climb or stand on an unsafe stool or ladder to reach high shelves in closets or cupboards. Do not lift or push any heavy objects that weigh more than the weight restrictions your doctor has imposed during your pregnancy.

Do not overdo it during the nesting phase. You may feel like you have energy to spare, but you don't want to get sore and overly tired. Make a list of what you would like to accomplish and then pace yourself and do just what you're comfortable with each day. It is important during the last few weeks of pregnancy not to become overly tired or sore from cleaning and organizing. You never know when the contractions may start and you won't want to be exhausted and sore when you go to the hospital for the delivery. Alternate heavier cleaning days with days of fun projects such as washing and folding baby clothes or starting your baby's scrapbook with the nursery photos you have taken.

Organize your finances. During your nesting time you will also want to get your bills and finances organized. The last thing you want to do is come home from the hospital with monthly bills to deal with. Send out monthly payments and utility bills in advance if you can. Take care of banking as much in advance as possible unless your husband, significant other or a friend has been asked in advance to help you with this task. For the first few days after you are home from the hospital, your focus will be on taking care of your baby. It won't be a good time to deal with bills. You'll be amazed at how difficult it may be to find an uninterrupted hour to work on bills, and if you do have uninterrupted time, you'll probably want to sleep!

Arrange for pet and plant care. If you have pets or houseplants that will need to be cared for during your hospital stay and for a few days after you return from the hospital, make these arrangements a few weeks ahead of time. Make sure you have a Plan B, in case Plan A does not work out at the last minute. Write out clear instructions for the person who is taking care of your pet and have plenty of pet food and pet supplies on hand.

Stock the kitchen. Stock the house with nonperishable groceries and some fresh veggies and fruit so you won't have to go to the market right away upon your arrival home. Consider convenient foods such as healthy prepared soups, yogurt and fruit, and healthy sandwich makings. Remember that when you bring your baby home from the hospital, particularly if you are nursing, you will need to drink a lot of water. If you do not have safe drinking water from the tap, stock up on bottled water and non-caffeine herbal teas that are safe to drink during nursing. If friends and family members have not volunteered to bring meals or organized a team from church or neighbors to bring meals, stock the freezer with a few frozen dishes that can be popped into the oven for easy dinners.

Unless you are really environmentally opposed to using paper plates and cups, consider stocking up on them and using them for the first few days after you arrive home from the hospital. Even if you have someone at home to help you out, they will have more important things to do than load and unload the dishwasher. Keep in mind that any practical thing you can do for convenience during those first few days after the baby's arrival, will be very helpful.

Install the baby car seat. A few weeks before you go to the hospital, install the baby car seat in your car. Be sure that you or whoever installs the seat follows all installation instructions. Check several times to make sure the seat is securely and correctly installed. In some areas, you can have the car seat checked for safety and correct installation at the local police department or fire department. When you install the car seat, put a couple of water-proof pads in the glove compartment of the car to put on the seat for the ride to the hospital, in case your water breaks. You can buy the pads at any drug store. The pads will come in handy for your bed upon return home from the hospital.

Arrange for a backup driver to the hospital. If there is any possibility that your partner may not be able to be reached to drive you to the hospital when you need to go, arrange for a dependable back-up driver. It is always good to have someone else "on call" just in case your car failed or something happened at the last minute to change your plans for getting to the hospital. Of course, if the situation demands it, you can call 911 at the hospital and get an ambulance for transport to the hospital. Ambulance transport is very expensive and in high demand for emergency situations, so should be used only in emergency situations or if you have no other option.

To a baby, it does not make any difference if it is three o'clock in the morning or mid-afternoon when it is time for them to make their debut into the world. Do not be shocked if your baby decides to be born late at night or very early in the morning. For this reason, you need to keep plenty of gasoline in the car at all times to get to the hospital and back home again. This is especially true if you live in a small town where gas stations do not stay open all night, or if you live several miles from the hospital. Even if gas stations are open, you will not want the major inconvenience of the driver stopping on your way to the hospital.

Home Check List

The home check list will vary for each individual. This is a general list that can be used to help you cover all of the basics.

- ✓ You have sent the bills for the month or have prepared them for mailing or paying online.
- ✓ You have arranged for the mail to be picked up or held at post office if you are going to be in the hospital for a few days.
- ✓ Arrangements for pet care have been made for while you are away at the hospital. (Also a back-up plan has been made in case Plan A falls through.)
- ✓ The kitchen has been stocked with healthy convenience foods, paper goods, and staples.
- ✓ You have completed your cleaning and organizing list.
- ✓ The baby car seat has been correctly installed in the car and double-checked for safety.
- ✓ You have put two water proof pads in the car to cover the seat on the way to the hospital, in case your water breaks while traveling to the hospital.

Pack Your Hospital Bag

When it is time to go to the hospital, the only thing you'll be thinking about is getting there on time. Every new mom seems to worry that she won't reach the hospital before the baby is born. Most often, there is no need to worry, as you have already planned out your hospital route and have timed how long it takes you to get there. Even if you have plenty of time to pack your hospital bag, you won't be focused on what you need to take with you. It is best to pack your hospital bag a few weeks ahead of time so you do not forget anything or have to send someone back to your home to look for what you need.

Before you pack your bag, check with the hospital to see what is provided free of charge for your use. Some hospitals charge for everything you use while there, including personal items such as a tube of hand cream or a box of tissue. Other hospitals provide some personal items without adding them to your hospital bill. If you are not certain about what is provided, it is best to take your own personal items. If the hospital charges you for any extra items, the price they charge will be considerably higher than what it would cost you to purchase privately.

Hospital Bag Check List

You'll need to pack items for yourself and your baby for the hospital stay and your trip home. Your partner will also need to have their bag packed and ready to go for their stay at the hospital with you.

Women who have already had their babies often bemoan the bad hospital food and they advice taking good snacks and plenty of cash for ordering take-out food, rather than eating hospital food. Hospital cafeterias vary greatly, some having good food, while others serve highly institutional, tasteless bland food. You may be able to find out what type of food your hospital has by visiting the cafeteria ahead of time, or asking friends or family members who have been in that hospital. Keep in mind that friends and family who stop by for visits want to help out and would probably be happy to bring good food if you request it.

Mommy's Hospital Bag

- ✓ Hospital admission papers, insurance card, and Identification
- ✓ Birthing plan, signed by you and your husband
- ✓ Calendar so you can write down pediatrician and doctor visits
- ✓ List of family and friends with phone numbers to call after baby is born, or a phone number to call the person that you have assigned to call everyone else
- ✓ Clothes for going home. Keep in mind that you probably won't want to wear your pre-pregnant jeans or tighter clothes even if you can fit into them. You'll want to wear lose clothing as when you first go home you will still "look" pregnant. Baggy pants with

a draw string waist and a baggy top are ideal. If you are nursing, you may want to take a nursing or button-down top with you.

✓ Nightgown and robe (a couple of nursing gowns or tops with button fronts if you are nursing your baby)

✓ Nursing bras and plenty of nursing pads if you are nursing your baby. Take a daytime nursing bra and one or two for sleeping.

✓ Several pair of underwear (consider packing underwear a size larger than you normally wear and briefs even if you normally wear bikinis, to adjust for and keep the large maxi-pads in place. If you have a cesarean you would want lose underwear that is higher up on the waist so the elastic does not rest on the stitches.)

✓ Toothpaste and toothbrush

✓ Bath soap and personal toiletries

✓ Shampoo and conditioner

✓ Several washcloths and a couple of towels. (Do not take white ones as they may get tossed into hospital laundry by accident.)

✓ Makeup (if you wear makeup and want to have it on for pictures or when visitors come.)

✓ House slippers or thick socks

✓ Lip balm—your lips will be dry during labor

✓ Water bottle with your name written on it

✓ Lotion or hand cream

✓ Breast ointment if you are breastfeeding, to put on sore nipples if necessary

✓ Maximum size feminine pads (though the hospital will have them available)

✓ Hair dryer and other hair-styling tools, including barrettes or headbands, etc.

✓ Baby book so nurse can "footprint" the baby in your book

✓ Guest book for registering visitors and noting their gifts while in hospital

✓ Birth announcements and thank you cards to work on while baby is sleeping

✓ Camera and/or video recorder with batteries

✓ Your favorite CD to relax by

✓ A few magazines or a book, a crossword puzzle book, or quiet hobby supplies to occupy your time when the baby is sleeping.

Baby's Hospital Bag

✓ Going home clothes. Some moms like to choose special dress-up clothes for baby's homecoming as this event is often captured in photos and/or on video. Other moms prefer that the baby be comfortable in their sleeper.

✓ Diaper bag with standard items for short trip home

✓ Going home blanket (While in the hospital, the hospital will supply receiving blankets.)

✓ The hospital will put disposable diapers on your baby while at the hospital. If you object to this, talk to the nursing staff ahead of time and arrange to use your own cloth diapers while at the hospital. Of course, you and Dad will probably be held responsible for all diapering if you choose to use cloth diapers, so you'll want to take a diaper pail or some sort of system for taking care of diapers.

Daddy's Hospital Bag

✓ Change of clothes

✓ Clean socks and underwear

✓ Something comfortable for sleeping in

✓ Personal toiletries and shaver (Dad needs to look good for the hospital pics too!)

✓ Camera and/or video recorder with batteries

✓ List of phone numbers for calling family members and close friends

✓ House slippers

✓ Identification

✓ Books or magazines to read

Double-Check the Nursery

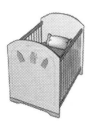 You've probably had the baby's nursery ready for weeks, but one final check before you go to the hospital won't hurt anything. Go back over your check list to make sure you have everything you really need and to see that the nursery is well organized.

Babies are simple bundles of joy, with simple needs. Of course, shopping for babies is great fun when the budget allows it, and there may be many extra items that you want to have available for convenience. As your baby grows, their needs will change. But here is a basic list of the basic things you'll need when you bring your baby home from the hospital.

Nursery Checklist

- ✓ Safe, comfortable crib, co-sleeper, or bassinette with firm mattress. (Double check that crib meets safety standards.)
- ✓ Clean, non-flammable bedding: 3 or 4 crib and bassinette sheets, crib bumper pads if you choose to use them, 5 or 6 receiving blankets, 3-4 warm blankets or wraps, depending on the season
- ✓ Five to seven season-appropriate sleepers
- ✓ Five to seven undershirts or onesies
- ✓ Six to eight pairs of socks or booties
- ✓ Three to four sets of mitts for baby's hands to keep them from scratching their face
- ✓ Three to four simple cotton knit hats to keep head warm
- ✓ Warm blanket sleeper for outdoor wear if it is winter in cold climate
- ✓ Diaper changing pad or table, and area to store diapers and changing supplies
- ✓ About three dozen diapers—cloth or disposable
- ✓ About six diaper covers if cloth diapers are used
- ✓ Diaper pins if cloth diapers are used
- ✓ Diaper wipes, cotton pads or balls, or a lot of soft washcloths that you can sanitize
- ✓ Diaper pail and deodorizing system
- ✓ Baby nail scissors or clippers
- ✓ Nasal aspirator
- ✓ Thermometer
- ✓ Baby washcloths for baths
- ✓ Baby tub or mat for bathing
- ✓ If you are not nursing, you'll need baby bottles, bottle brush, a system for sterilizing bottles, bottle nipples, formula
- ✓ Soft bristle baby brush and comb

✓ A night light with soft light so you can see what you are doing when you change or feed the baby during the night.

✓ A comfortable chair or rocker for relaxing while feeding the baby.

✓ A dresser or cubby system for holding baby's blankets, sleepers, undershirts, etc.

✓ Burping pads (clean cloth diapers can be used for this)

✓ Breast pump if you intend to nurse your newborn and will be leaving him/her with others while you work or go out

✓ Infant carrier (most large strollers now come with removal infant carriers that can be strapped into the car seat)

✓ Car seat that meets safety standards

Other Items that can be Useful

This list will grow and change as baby grows. Here are some basic items that are not necessities, but are useful during first few months:

✓ Baby swing

✓ Stroller

✓ Nursing pillow

✓ Sling or front/back pack for carrying baby close to you

✓ Pacifier for a little later

Test Drive the Hospital Route

You've talked with your doctor and you have determined at what point you should leave for the hospital. A few weeks before your due date, it is good to drive the route to the hospital and see how long it takes you to get there. Take the drive during different times of the day. Figure out the best route to take based on traffic, number of stop signs and traffic lights etc. If your baby is due during the winter months and you live in an area where there is snow and ice, allow extra time for safe driving to the hospital. During the last few weeks of your pregnancy, keep plenty of gas in the car to ensure that you do not have to stop for a refill on the way to the hospital.

Classes

Many women prefer to do their own research regarding pregnancy, child birth and infant care. They read books on the topics and search the Internet for articles. They talk to other women who have already had children. But sometimes having an instructor can be beneficial. There are various classes for pregnant women and new moms, including:

➢ **Lamaze** childbirth education that emphasizes breathing techniques during labor.

➢ **Bradley** childbirth classes that emphasize drug-free childbirth.

➢ **Exercise classes** for pregnant women such as yoga and water aerobics or walking groups. At the very least, learn to do Kegel exercises which you can do anywhere at any time to help strengthen the pelvic floor muscles and make your delivery much easier.

➢ **Breastfeeding classes** that encourage moms to breastfeed, and inform and prepare new moms for breastfeeding. (You can visit Le Leche at http://www.llli.org/WebUS.html to find a local Le Leche group.)

➢ **Infant care classes** are often offered through county health clinics, birthing centers and parenting groups.

3

IT'S TIME! HOSPITAL AND DELIVERY

When Should I Go to the Hospital?

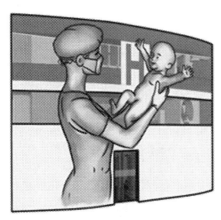

It is natural for first-time moms to be anxious about getting to the hospital when they first start feeling contractions. If you have talked to women who have already had babies, they assure you that you'll *just know* when it is really time to go to the hospital. Still, you may be afraid you won't leave for the hospital on time. To help relieve anxiety, talk with your doctor about when you should go to the hospital after your contractions start. Some doctors prefer that their patients wait at home as long as possible, while others prefer for their patients to arrive with ample time for check-in and prep. Often, the doctor will recommend the 411 Rule. This means you'll time your contractions and go to the hospital when the contractions are four minutes apart, lasting for one minute, for a period of one hour.

> **411 Rule: Contractions are four minutes apart, lasting one minute each, for one hour.**

It is important to understand the difference between Braxton Hicks and "real" contractions that start the delivery of your baby. Braxton Hicks are real contractions that usually start sometime during the second trimester, but they do not cause dilation or effacing of the cervix to move along the birth. For this reason they are sometimes called "fake contractions," even though they may not feel "fake" at all. They can be triggered by stimulation as simple as touching your stomach or the baby being active. Braxton Hicks actually help prepare your uterus for the birth.

First time moms may feel like the Braxton Hicks are quite painful, but compared to the delivery room contractions, they are usually fairly mild. However, some women do experience quite painful Braxton Hicks. Braxton Hicks usually only last a few seconds and may come and go. Sometimes they will return a short time later, and often they won't return for weeks. If you have Braxton Hicks and are not sure whether you are in labor, call your doctor and discuss what is happening. It is always better to be on the safe side. Also, if you think you are just having Braxton Hicks but they become extremely painful, call your doctor.

If you go to the hospital as soon as your labor starts, the delivery nurse may decide not to admit you if you are still obviously several hours from delivery time. The policy at many hospitals is not to admit for delivery until the cervix is dilated to at least three or four centimeters. The nurse may suggest that you go back home or wait in the hospital lobby until you are closer to your delivery time. The exception would be if you live several miles from the hospital and it would take significant time to travel back home and then back to the hospital; or if you have other special reasons for wanting to wait at the hospital until you are deeper into your labor. Speak up if you feel it is best to remain at the hospital, but keep in mind that you will probably be more comfortable laboring at home rather than waiting around at the hospital.

Hospital Registration and Check-In

Your hospital registration should have previously been completed as per your doctor's instructions and hospital policy. By this point, your doctor has probably given you hospital admission instructions. If your hospital paperwork is not completed, you will probably have to fill out the required forms before you go to the delivery room. If your paperwork is completed when you arrive at the hospital, check in at the birthing center or maternity station and a nurse will direct you. Be sure to have your photo identification with you when you go to the hospital.

The nurse will ask you to explain what is happening with your body and ask questions about the timing of your contractions, whether your water has broken, how you are feeling, if anything unusual has happened, etc. The nurse will probably put their hand on your stomach to get an indication of the baby's position, and also take your blood pressure level, pulse rate and temperature.

Preparing For Delivery

Once you have been admitted to the hospital and the room is being prepared for delivery, the nurse will ask you about your birth plan. Be honest and speak up about your wishes and present your written birth plan if you have one. (See worksheet for birth plan at the end of the chapter.) Your baby's delivery is a very special and personal time for you and your partner; you need to be sure your doctor and the hospital staff know and follow your birthing wishes. Your written birth plan will be very helpful to the staff. The birth plan will make your birthing philosophy known, as well as instruct on such issues as whether you want to have a perennial shave, have an episiotomy, a natural delivery without medication, or an epidural, whether you want to lie down or be upright during labor, who can be in the room with you during the delivery, and your wish for other delivery procedures.

The nurses will set up the delivery station and equipment. They will prepare a birthing place for you, set up a warming station for the baby, and set up all of the monitoring equipment. You will be attached to machines that monitor your contractions and the baby's heartbeat throughout your labor stages. Good nurses usually explain what they are doing and what equipment is being used as they prepare you for delivery. If the nurse does not explain, ask any questions you have.

Usually, the hospital orderlies or nurses will set up a bed for your partner so they can rest and stay in the room with you overnight. Your partner can be very helpful during the delivery process and should be informed and aware of what is going on. Help prepare your partner and anyone else who will be in the delivery room for what will happen in the delivery room. This will minimize their fear and optimize their ability to help out as needed. Dad will probably be quite nervous, but it is advisable not to have any other fearful or nervous person in the delivery hospital staff. Anyone who remains in the delivery room should be alert to what is going on and aware that the priority is yours and the baby's safety at all times.

In the Delivery Room

If you talk to ten women who have given birth, each will probably share a different delivery room experience. No two deliveries are exactly the same. So, if you have heard a lot of stories about bad delivery experiences—block those stories from your mind and remember that this is *your* delivery. There is no doubt about it—you will work hard in the delivery room, and yes, the pain will be substantial. But the entire time you are laboring, you'll be motivated by the fact that you'll get to see your newborn baby soon! Your delivery room experience can be a positive one if you maintain a positive attitude and keep your mind on your end goal.

The most important thing to remember when you go into the delivery room is, to try your best to relax. Even though you may be eager to get on with the delivery, sometimes hours and hours can pass from the time you enter the delivery room until your baby is born. Be prepared to go the distance and do not be in such a hurry to get to the finish line. Anxiety about getting to the finish line will create tension and stress, which is not good for Mommy or Baby. Relax.

The delivery room nurses will set up machines so they (and you) can monitor the length and frequency of your contractions and the baby's heart beat. They will also insert an IV into the vein on your hand. If you have requested an epidural, the anesthesiologist or your doctor will administer it at the right time.

The nurses will also check you to see how dilated the cervix is. This may seem annoying and quite uncomfortable, but it is necessary. The nurses understand that they are inconveniencing you and making you feel more uncomfortable during your contractions. Try to be considerate of them, but if you get snappy or cross, do not be afraid that they'll be offended. Even the kindest, most well-mannered woman can easily lose it during labor!

The Labor Stages and Delivery

Some women are in labor for only a few hours, while others are in labor for twenty hours or more. Again, every delivery is different. There are different stages of labor. Understanding each stage will give you confidence that you are progressing toward your baby's birth at each stage. It also helps if your partner and those who are going to be in the delivery room with you understand the stages of labor.

> **Latent Labor** is also often called early labor. This early stage of labor can last anywhere from around two to three hours to around twelve or more hours. First-time moms usually have longer early labor than women who have given birth before. When the early stage of labor begins, call your doctor and let her/him know that you are in early labor. Your doctor will advise you on what to do next. Usually the doctor's advice will be to try to walk slowly during this time to keep the labor going, but do not go to the hospital until you are approaching the end of the early labor stage.
>
> During the early labor stage, the cervix dilates up to about 3 centimeters. Your contractions will occur about every five to twenty minutes and last 30 to 45 seconds each time. You may lose your mucous plug during this stage or have a "bloody show." But do not worry if this does not happen because you may have already lost the mucous plug hours or days before the early labor stage.
>
> **Active Labor** is usually the most painful part of the delivery process. During this stage, the contractions are more intense

and painful and will occur about every three to five minutes and last 45 seconds to one minute each. The cervix will dilate from three to seven centimeters during this stage. As the contractions intensify, you may decide to have an epidural. Your doctor or anesthesiologist will administer the epidural. The epidural should help you relax and considerably ease the pain.

> **Transitional Labor** is the shortest labor stage, during which the cervix will dilate all the way to ten centimeters in preparation for the birth. The transition stage usually lasts less than an hour, but the contractions are very intense and occur every two to three minutes and last about 60 to 90 seconds each. Focused breathing during this stage is essential for helping to cope with the pain.

> **Pushing** is the stage of labor that a new mom usually thinks of when she thinks of labor. At this stage a mom knows her hard work and enduring of pain has paid off and she is getting very close to being able to finally see her precious baby. This encourages the mom and she exhibits a final blast of energy that she did not know she had in her!

During the pushing stage, contractions occur about every three to five minutes and become a little less intense. You will feel a strong urge to push as hard as you can to get the baby out, but you will need to listen to and follow the instructions given by the doctor or nurse for pushing.

Your doctor or the nurse will keep you informed of the progress of the baby. You'll be so delighted when you hear them say the baby's head is crowning. At that point, you'll know you are very close to completion! The pushing stage of delivery usually last between thirty to ninety minutes.

The nurses will probably wait until it is close to the time for the baby to be born before they call in your doctor. Do not be nervous that the doctor won't make it on time. Birthing nurses are very experienced at knowing how close you are to giving birth, and will call your doctor ahead of time to make sure the doctor is standing by for your delivery. The doctor almost always arrives on time. And, if something should happen where the doctor does not make it on time, do not panic. You'll be in good hands with competent delivery room nurses.

Episiotomy

Doctors try to avoid doing episiotomies, but if during your labor they feel the opening needs to be larger for the baby to be born, he/she will do an episiotomy to help avoid natural tearing. The episiotomy is a procedure where the doctor makes a cut in the area between the vagina and perineum, allowing for a larger opening for the baby's head to pass through. The doctor will numb the area before making the cut, and with everything else that is going on, mom may not even feel the procedure. After the baby is born and the placenta has been expelled, the doctor will stitch the cut with dissolvable stitches. The doctor or nurse will give clear instructions for the care of the stitches to avoid infection.

The Baby is Born, Now What?

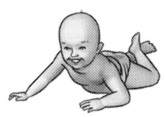

The Afterbirth

After the baby is delivered, you will feel more contractions. Your body will expel the placenta and the fetal membranes. Doctors and nurses often refer to this as the *afterbirth*. Expelling the placenta may happen within minutes after delivery or it may take up to an hour. The placenta is about one-fifth the size of the baby and is expelled into a small hospital tub.

Some women want to keep the placenta. Your doctor or nurse will ask what your preference is. While it is beyond the scope of this book to explain, there is a recent development of mothers who have just birthed their babies, ingesting the placenta for immune system and nutritional properties.

Your doctor may give you Pitocin (oxytocin) after the placenta is delivered, to help your uterus contract so the bleeding will slow down. Sometimes the medication is given as an injection, but most often it is included in the IV fluids you have been given. Natural alternatives to Pitocin are externally massaging the uterus or letting your baby immediately suck at your breast to stimulate contractions.

Your doctor will check your perennial area for any tears. The tears and episiotomy cut (if you had an episiotomy) will be stitched. You'll be cleaned up and will be put on a pad, as the bleeding will continue. Nurses will explain to you when you may shower, how to take care of your stitches, etc. The nurses will continue to monitor you.

The Nurses Will Take Care of the Baby

While the doctor is finishing the after-birth details, the nurses will take care of your baby. The baby's nose and mouth will be suctioned to remove mucous. The umbilical cord will be clamped and you or Dad will have the chance to cut the umbilical cord. If neither of you wants to cut the cord, your doctor or the nurse will do it. You should decide this ahead of time, as everything will happen quickly in the delivery room once the baby is born. In fact, it is not uncommon for women to say that they do not remember the details of their first time in the delivery room.

The baby will be given a shot of Vitamin K to help clot the blood, and antibiotic ointment will be put in the eyes to help avoid infection. Baby will be measured, weighed, and the foot prints will be taken. The nurses will put an identification band on your baby's wrist and ankle. The baby will be washed and the umbilical cord stem will be cleaned. Once the baby is clean and diapered, he/she will be delivered to mom and dad to hold. It may seem like hours pass from the time that the baby is delivered until he/she is brought to you, but in reality, it all happens fairly quickly. The delivery room will be buzzing during this time, with nurses continuing to take care of you and other nurses taking care of your baby.

Bonding With Your Baby

When the nurse brings your baby to you, it will be a highly emotional moment that you and dad have been waiting for and will never forget. You are a MOM now and you are holding your baby! This will be a bonding moment for you, baby and dad. It may not seem real to you at first, but after you have had some rest, all that has transpired will sink in and you'll have plenty of time to get used to being a mommy.

Allow yourself plenty of time to hold your baby while you have extra help with him/her at the hospital. This may mean that you have to limit visitors. Friends and family will be eager to see your baby, but their visiting should not interfere with you and your partner taking care of and getting to know your baby.

Feeding Your Baby

If you're breastfeeding your baby, your milk won't instantly come in, but your baby will still nurse right away on the colostrum. The colostrum contains immune-system-building and antibacterial properties to help protect your baby, and the nutrients your baby needs for a healthy start in life. Let your baby nurse as soon as possible and as frequently as they want to on the colostrum, as it comes in slowly and your baby will need to "eat" frequently.

Your breast milk will come in within the first three to four days after the baby is delivered. (Your milk will come in even if you do not breastfeed your baby; so be prepared with a sturdy bra and nursing shields to prevent leakage.) You will probably already be home from the hospital by the time your milk comes in, but by then your baby would have learned how to nurse under the watchful eyes of the hospital nurses and your doctor.

If you are bottle feeding baby formula to your baby, the hospital will provide pre-made bottles of formula while you are at the hospital. In most instances, the mother has a choice of which formula the baby will be given and what type of bottle nipple will be used. This is something for you to decide ahead of time. Whatever formula you start the baby on, is the one you will probably want to remain with after you leave the hospital; unless there is a reason that your baby does not do well on a particular formula.

Just as with breastfeeding, your newborn will need to learn how to suck at the bottle nipple and will need some practice. Do not worry if your baby does not instantly know how to suck the nipple. He/she will catch on soon enough. The hospital nurses or pediatrician will monitor your baby to make sure he/she is getting enough formula.

While at the hospital, your baby will get a PKU, which is a prick on the heel. The PKU tests the baby's ability to digest protein. The baby will also be tested for galactosemia, hemoglobinopathy, hypothyroidism, and adrenal hyperplasia. Do not be afraid to ask precise questions about what the pediatrician and nurses are doing with your baby. You have a right to be informed, and they won't mind explaining what is going on.

While in the hospital, you will have the opportunity to hold and breastfeed your baby. You will probably be able to have the baby in your room with you all the time if you want to. But if you need the nurses to take the baby to the nursery or help with the baby while you get some sleep, do not be afraid to ask.

Going Home

After the birth, your hospital stay will be fairly short. The average hospital stay for vaginal births is 48 hours if there are no complications with mom or baby. However, sometimes new moms are released after 24 hours if all is well. If you have a Cesarean birth, your hospital stay will probably be four to six days.

Most hospitals have strict discharge policies. Forms of all kinds have to be signed to release the hospital of liability and to ensure them that you have been instructed on how to take care of yourself after you leave the hospital. Make sure you know what you are signing before you sign anything. If you are tired and not thinking clearly when asked to sign a form, ask your partner to read the form out loud to you, or ask the hospital staff or nurse to bring the papers back to you at a later time. Keep all of your hospital paperwork so you can refer back to it if needed.

Usually, the hospital will send you home with various "gifts" that come from baby product manufacturers. The gifts may include everything from samples of baby bath products to diaper bags to disposable diapers. If you are bottle feeding your baby, you will probably be sent home with pre-made formula bottles and other formula. The idea is for you to try out these products and hopefully buy them once the samples are gone.

Your hospital staff will probably offer you the option of having your baby's picture taken while at the hospital. This is usually outsourced to a photographer or photography company, so the prices for the photos vary. In most cases, you will be given a form to fill out and the photo shoot will be scheduled. You will be sent the photos in the mail. You may also hire your own photographer to come to the hospital for a photo shoot. However, keep in mind that your baby is not interested in anyone's schedule but their own. If they decide to eat or poop their diaper or cry during the photo shoot, there really isn't anything that you can do about it. If you want professionally shot photos of your newborn, it may be easier to have the photographer come to your home or for you to go to their studio at your convenience.

When you leave the hospital, the nurse or an orderly may make sure your baby is properly strapped into a safe baby carrier seat (hospital policies vary.) In this economy, the expense of having a baby can be overwhelming. If you cannot afford to purchase a safe baby carrier seat that straps into your car before your baby is born, contact local social organizations and ask for help with getting a car seat. If you do not find help through a social organization, contact your local sheriff department and hospital and tell them your situation. There are some service organizations that provide safety car seats for parents who cannot afford to buy one.

You have been through a lot over the past few days and now you are finally on your way home with your newborn! The joy is just beginning!

My Birth Plan Worksheet

Besides delivery room staff and my doctor, I'd like the following people to be allowed in the delivery room with me.

1.
2.
3.
4.
5.

After the birth, I want the following people to be allowed in my room as soon as possible after the baby is washed, diapered, and available to see.

I want _____ to video or take pictures during the labor and delivery, following these instructions:

I want the following music played during labor and delivery:

Labor Preferences: (Check all that apply)

- o I do want a pre-labor perineal shave.
- o I do not want a pre-labor perineal shave.
- o I want my partner to stay with me at all times.
- o I want my partner involved in every decision that needs to be made.

o   I want to make all of the decisions on my own without my partner's involvement.

o   I do not want my baby to be taken from my presence or my partner's presence, except in event of emergency.

o   I do not want any medical students, residents, or other hospital personnel present during labor and delivery. (Doctor and nurses are exceptions, of course.)

o   I do not mind if medical students, residents, or other hospital personnel are present during labor and delivery.

o   I'd like to be in an upright position during delivery.

o   I'd like to lie down on my back or side during delivery.

o   If available, I'd like to use a birthing stool.

o   If available, I'd like to use a birthing chair.

o   If available, I'd like to use a birthing pool.

o   I do not want an IV. I would prefer to stay hydrated with drinking clear fluids.

o   I want to have a heparin or saline lock

o   I want continuous electronic fetal monitoring.

o   I want only intermittent electronic fetal monitoring; unless there is a problem that creates need for constant monitoring.

o   I want to be able to walk around as much as I want, without being scolded to stay in bed. Explanation:

o   For pain management, I'd like to use bath/shower. Explanation:

o   For pain management, I'd like to have my partner give me a massage. Explanation:

o   For pain management, I'd like to use breathing techniques. Explanation:

o   For pain management, I'd like to use hot/cold therapy. Explanation:

o   For pain management, I'd like to use medication. Explanation:

o I do not want to have any pain medication. If I change my mind I will ask for it. Explanation:

o If I want pain medication, I want a regional analgesia (epidural or spinal block) Explain:

o Systemic medication. Explain:

o I do not want Pitocin. I prefer the following alternative methods for causing uterine contractions and reduction of bleeding after the delivery:

o I want to feed my baby on schedule. Explain schedule:

o I want to feed my baby on demand. Explain:

o I want to have my baby boy circumcised at the hospital. Instructions:

o I do not want to have my baby boy circumcised.

o I do not want to have an episiotomy.

o I do want an episiotomy if the doctor feels it is necessary.

o I want to breastfeed exclusively.

o I want to breastfeed and formula bottle feed my baby. Explain:

o   I do not want my baby to receive any formula.

o   I do not want my baby to be given any sugar water.

o   I do not want my baby to be given a pacifier.

o   I prefer to be discharged from the hospital as soon as possible.

o   I do not have help at home and prefer to stay at the hospital for the longest time possible.

Other wishes and instructions:

Signed: _____ Date: _____

4

TAKING CARE OF YOURSELF
AFTER DELIVERY

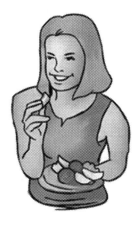 When you get home from the hospital with your newborn, the reality that you are a parent and that your newborn is totally dependent on you for everything he/she needs, may hit you hard. You may suddenly feel lost—as though you are all alone with the responsibility for this new baby and are not sure you know what to do. This is a normal feeling. Even doctors and nurses say they have these same feelings when they arrive home with their newborns; even though they are well informed about taking care of a newborn baby.

Take a few deep breaths and put everything in perspective. Every day millions of babies are born around the world, and every day millions of first-time moms do what comes naturally to them—they take care of their infants. They nourish them with breast milk or with formula, they diaper them and keep them clean, they protect them from anything that could harm them, they hold them close and love them. If they sense something is wrong, they follow their motherly instinct and get medical help. Really, it's all very simple and you are very capable!

Also take comfort in the fact that you can always call your pediatrician for any medical/health related questions and you can call on trusted friends and family members for advice too. With the Internet at your fingertips, you can find the answer to just about any question that pops up. Just be sure you are getting solid, accurate information from reputable sources. If you doubt that information is reliable, do not trust it. It's too risky.

Before the baby is born, talk with your partner about shared responsibilities for the baby and managing the household. When you get home from the hospital, let your partner know that you definitely need their help and what you expect of them. Dad can do everything that mom can do for the baby, except breastfeed, of course. Taking care of baby is a good way for dad to bond with the baby and overcome the common fear of making a mistake or accidentally hurting baby. It won't take dad very long to see that baby won't break and is easily handled, and he will enjoy spending time with his baby.

Be patient with dad while he is learning to help. Do not nag and constantly correct him. This will make him feel inadequate and left out of the picture. He'll catch on soon with just a little gentle coaching from you. You may be tempted to laugh at his first attempt at changing a diaper, but be kind and praise him for helping out. Remember, this baby thing is new for him too! And he may be a lot more afraid of it than you are, though he may not be willing to admit it.

You may also want to enlist the help of a trusted friend, your mother, or a sister. If you do enlist outside help, make sure you do not end up feeling like you need to entertain or host the person. They are there to help—let them help. While the visiting will be nice, you should not feel like you are "hosting" your helper and need to accommodate them. That would put added stress on you during a time when you will need to focus on your new baby and recovering from the delivery.

Taking Care of Your Body

After birth, you will be able to take better care of your baby if you also take great care of yourself. Follow your doctor's orders for taking it easy and giving your body time to recuperate after birthing your baby. Though giving birth is a natural process, it is still a tremendous process for your body to have gone through!

Within two to three days of getting home, your breasts may become engorged with milk, and will be tender and swollen. Wear nursing pads to prevent leakage. You will also need to continue to wear sanitary napkins to collect vaginal discharge. You will continue to feel contractions, particularly when breast feeding. The vaginal area will be sore for several days and walking won't be without a little pain. Follow your doctor's orders in caring for after birth stitches. A warm sitz bath can relieve the stinging and itching in the stitches area.

Keep all of the medical care advice and warning instructions given to you at the hospital. Do not hesitate to call your doctor if you have any alarming symptoms or if you have any unusual issues that you do not understand. As always, it is better to be safe than to be sorry!

Get Sleep Whenever You Can

You have heard all the jokes about never sleeping again once the baby is born, and granted, sleep will be a rare commodity for the first few weeks after your baby's birth—but you must do your best to sleep whenever you can, even if it is a short 20-minute nap. If you have to choose between washing the dishes and getting a thirty-minute nap while baby is sleeping, always take the nap! You can always get someone else to help out with dishes, but no one else can sleep for you!

Getting rest whenever you can will keep you from pushing yourself to the point of being frazzled. You'll be happier and enjoy your baby more if you are not exhausted. It will be much easier for you and your partner to cope with and adjust to your new lifestyle with a baby if you are not tired. Even if you are breastfeeding your baby, if you are suffering from severe sleep deprivation you can express breast milk and let your partner give the baby a middle-of-the-night bottle or two. If your baby insists on staying awake all night and sleeping all day, do your best to sleep as much as possible during the day until your baby starts to sleep at night.

Continue a Healthy Diet

Hopefully, during your pregnancy you maintained a healthy diet with lots of fresh fruit and vegetables, whole grains, lean meat, and dairy products.

It is important to keep up the healthy diet after the birth, so you can heal, have plenty of energy, stay healthy and produce plenty of milk for your baby if you are breastfeeding. Maintaining a healthy diet will also help you get back to your normal weight faster, too. If you are a nursing mom, it is imperative for you to always drink even more water than usual every day. Stay well hydrated! As always, try to avoid caffeine and sugary, fatty foods; particularly if you are nursing.

Exercise!

It may seem difficult to find the time, but another great way to take care of yourself is to start exercising as soon as your doctor allows it. This will probably be about the time the baby is six weeks old. Before then, short walks in the sunshine and fresh air with your baby will help keep you mobile and provide you with a change of scenery to boost your mood and energy levels.

Baby Blues and Postpartum Depression

Pregnancy and birthing creates high levels of hormonal changes and fluctuations in a woman's body. You probably witnessed this when you first became pregnant and witnessed mood fluctuations; sometimes you felt like screaming or burst into tears for no reason at all. Remembering that can help you understand why during the happiest time of your life, you are having mixed feelings and even some feelings of sadness.

According to health care professionals, up to 80% of women experience emotional disturbances after giving birth. The disturbances can include feeling afraid, being upset, feeling sad, feeling like you are alone, and so forth. Women often feel guilty when they experience these feelings because they think they should only be having feelings of happiness and joy after the birth of their baby. Every new mom must understand that they should not feel guilty about the feelings they are having and that the baby blues will fade away.

The emotional disturbances can cause:

- Irritability

- Anxiety
- Lack of ability to sleep or sleep well
- Crying easily and for no particular reason
- Feelings of sadness
- Change in appetite
- Feeling like you are on the edge

The mixed emotions that cause these issues are often referred to as the "baby blues". Baby blues are quite normal and there is certainly no reason for the new mom to feel guilty for experiencing such emotions. Baby blues usually peak about three to five days after the baby is born and can last from two to three days to around two or three weeks. Baby blues are not considered an illness and do not need to be treated by a doctor unless you are blue for an extended period of time or severely so. The best treatment is to rest and sleep when you can and pace yourself to help avoid exhaustion. It is always more difficult to cope with strong emotions when you are tired. Also, talk to your partner about how you are feeling. If they are aware of the baby blues before you go to the hospital for delivery, they will understand what is happening when you are going through it and they can be helpful and supportive.

The new mom, who is taking good care of herself, should be able to continue to also take good care of her baby while going through the baby blues. However, if at any time you feel overwhelmed or feel like you cannot take care of your baby, you need to immediately seek professional help.

Postpartum Depression

Postpartum depression is not same as the baby blues. Even though they share many of the initial symptoms, postpartum depression is a more serious concern than baby blues. If a woman has had previous history of depression or she has had a very stressful pregnancy, she is more apt to experience postpartum depression. Postpartum depression can come on instantly, but in most cases it comes on gradually over a period of several months. It can affect the ability of the mom to function and to take care of her baby.

A mom who suffers from postpartum depression may feel intense feelings of guilt for not happy. She should not feel guilty or ashamed because these feelings are generated due to chemical changes going on in her body. Postpartum depression can be brought on by the rapid hormonal changes that occur during pregnancy and child birth, and other factors which a person has no control over. This, in addition to all the changes a woman's body goes through, her adjustment to caring for a newborn, and sleep deprivation can contribute to postpartum depression.

Below are the symptoms of postpartum depression. If you think you may be experiencing postpartum depression, talk to your doctor. He/she will be able to refer you to the appropriate medical professional.

Symptoms of Postpartum Depression

- Severely diminishing appetite, or even loss of it
- Fatigue that does not dissipate to some degree after resting and sleeping
- Insomnia
- Lack of joy
- Irritability over things that usually do not irritate you, or over everything
- Extreme mood swings for no apparent reason
- Prevailing sadness and melancholy
- Withdrawing from family and friends
- Detaching from baby/inability to bond with baby
- Feelings of inadequacy, shame, guilt, fear, helplessness
- Feelings of wanting to harm baby

The Medical Stuff

Your doctor and the delivery room nurses are very helpful with providing information on how to take care of your body after the delivery. Be sure you ask any questions you have before leaving the hospital and that you follow their instructions after you get home. Keep your follow-up appointments with your doctor, and do not hesitate to call your doctor in between appointments if you have any problems or questions.

Watch for Alarming Symptoms

Most women come home from the hospital and heal beautifully, with no problems at all. There is no reason to anticipate anything going wrong. With a little help from you, your body knows what to do and how to adjust back to its pre-pregnancy form.

However, there are certain things that can spell serious trouble for you after delivery, and you should be aware of the symptoms. Memorize this short caution-list. If you experience any of these things, call your doctor:

➤ Feelings that you want to hurt yourself or hurt your baby or completely neglect your baby
➤ Inability to function when your baby needs you
➤ Fever that is more than 100 degrees
➤ Heavy, bright red bleeding or passing large clots
➤ Severe cramps
➤ Increase of pain from episiotomy stitches/redness and swelling around stitches
➤ Pain when you urinate (Be sure to note the difference between pain in urinating and the mild burning that may occur when your urine comes in contact with episiotomy stitches.)

5

TAKING CARE OF YOUR NEWBORN

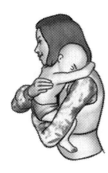

Obviously, your baby will have physical needs which you must be prepared to meet, such as feeding, diapering, and bathing. But your baby also has the need to feel secure, safe and loved. Your baby needs to feel an attachment to you. You are the bridge that takes your baby from the warmth and comfort of the womb to the big outside world. There are many ways you can help your baby feel safe and secure.

➤ Hold and cuddle your baby. Baby needs to feel your loving touch. Research shows that touching baby actually triggers hormones and helps fight diseases.

➤ Respond to your baby's needs for warmth, safety, food, and comfort. Do not ignore your baby or leave him/her wondering if the needs will be met.

➤ Talk to your baby often. It does not matter if the baby doesn't understand what you are saying. Your baby can hear your voice and recognize it as the voice he/she heard during the first nine months of their life in your womb. He/she can "connect" the voice with comfort and safety.

Whether breastfeeding or bottle feeding your baby, relax and sing softly to your baby while holding and feeding him/her. Do not put your baby in a baby carrier seat or the bassinette or crib to feed him/her, and never prop up the baby's bottle to feed him/her. Touch your baby often and hold him/

her close to you. Slings or infant front packs that allow you to carry your baby close to you while freeing your arms to do other things that you need to do are an excellent way to help your baby feel secure and attached.

If you have decided to return to work within a few weeks of your baby's birth, make sure your childcare provider understands the importance of nurturing your baby by talking to and holding him/her often. All too often, childcare providers for multiple children are overextended and cannot give an infant the individual time and attention they need. A tell-tale sign that your baby has been left in a car seat, baby swing, or crib for long periods of time is a flattened area in the back of baby's head. Babies that are not held and cuddled do not thrive as well.

Create Some Routines

Most babies seem more content when there is somewhat of a daily routine. This does not mean that you or the baby needs to be on a tight schedule. Little routines can be incorporated into whatever else you are doing. Even at a young age, babies seem to anticipate certain things at certain times or in a certain order. A sense of order can help them feel secure and sense that there is some sort of order in their world.

Sleeping

Your newborn will need to sleep about 14 to 18 hours per day during the first week or two of their life. After that, they will need to sleep about 12 to 16 hours per day. You may think that this would afford you plenty of time to sleep—but keep in mind that newborn babies only sleep for two to three hours at a time, during the day and during the night. People say that newborns get their days and nights confused, but infants do not know the difference between day and night. This means that your sleep is interrupted every few hours with feedings and diaper changes, and you never really get the deep restorative sleep that you need. It does not take long for you to become sleep deprived and very tired. It is important to try to find solutions that will allow you to get much needed sleep during the first few weeks after your baby is born.

> ➤ If you are not breastfeeding your baby, ask your partner to share the responsibility of night feedings. If you are breastfeeding, consider expressing breast milk to fill a bottle for your partner to give the baby so you can sleep through a few feedings. (Do a few test runs to make sure that your baby will be able to feed from the bottle.) On the "shift" that you are not on "baby duty", you may want to consider sleeping in another room so that when the baby wakes up, your sleep is not disturbed.

> ➤ Train yourself to take naps during the day when the baby sleeps. Do not be tempted to clean house, catch up on paperwork, or do other tasks instead. Even a 20-minute nap will help tremendously when you are sleep deprived. It will be easier for you to take care of your newborn without feeling overwhelmed if you are well rested. Playing "supermom" does not do you or your newborn any good.

> ➤ If your partner cannot share the responsibilities of night time feedings and diapering, you may need to call on a friend, sister, or your mother to help take care of the baby for a couple of hours during the day, while you sleep.

Fortunately, when your baby is about six to eight weeks old, it will be natural for them to start sleeping for longer periods at night. They will still need to eat during the night, but will need to eat at intervals of four to five hours instead of every two to three hours. By the time your baby is three to six months old, they will start to sleep for up to five or six hours at a time during the night. At this time, you can help your baby develop good sleeping habits.

Set Up and Follow a Bedtime Routine

Even at the early age of just three to four weeks old, within reason, your baby can start to adapt to whatever routine and pattern you set up, if you are consistent with it. Consistency is the key!

Take note of the times when your baby seems to sleep the longest periods of time. If he/she sleeps for a solid five hours from about eight o'clock in the evening, that will give you a clue that a good bedtime for your baby is eight o'clock. Make sure the time you choose to start your bedtime routine is *before* the baby gets overly tired. Once a newborn gets overly tired, they can have difficulty relaxing and going to sleep.

If you want your baby to sleep during certain hours, set up a routine to help them get quiet and relaxed about thirty to forty-five minutes before bed time. During quiet time, do not over stimulate your baby with noise or activity. Part of your bedtime routine may be a warm bath and/or massaging the baby's back to help him/her relax. You may enjoy reading out loud or singing to your baby while they drift off to sleep. (It does not matter if the baby "understands" the story or not, it is the sound and rhythm of your voice that the baby wants to hear.) You may want to play soft music or a recording of nature sounds such as ocean waves or chirping birds. You may want to rock your baby or put him/her in their crib, but always let the baby sleep in the same place so that he/she understands that when they are in that place, they are there to sleep.

Rocking your baby to sleep can be a special time for you. It is a wonderful bonding time and one that you will look forward to each evening. It gives you the time to cuddle your baby, study their precious face, and touch their soft skin. If you do choose to rock your baby in your arms, it is best to put her/him in their sleeping place just before they actually get to sleep, so they will learn to go to sleep without being held. Newborns usually go to sleep fairly quickly once they have had their bedtime routine, but your baby won't be a newborn forever. Once they are older, their stamina increases for having you rock them for hours before going to sleep.

Remember to be consistent and follow the same bedtime routine every single night. Choose the routine wisely, because whatever routine you choose is what the baby will expect (or demand) for many months to come. For instance if you rock the baby to sleep in your arms, that is what the baby will always expect from you, until a new routine is developed. As your baby grows and develops, you will need to adjust the routine if needed. Sometimes life changes will also dictate changing the bedtime routine. As an example, when Jill, an RN, returned to work when her baby boy was six months old, she worked a day time shift, but was switched to the night shift shortly thereafter. Jill had to change her baby's sleeping routine so she could nurse the baby and put him to bed before she had to leave for work every night.

Once you put your baby in the bassinet or crib, it is best not to take them back out, even if they start to whimper a bit. Gently pat their back and talk to them or sing to them to let them know that you are still with them and they will probably go ahead and sleep. If they do start to cry, it is safe to allow them to cry for a few minutes, if you are sure that they are well, are not hungry, are dry, and there are no other reasons for them to cry. It can be tremendously difficult and somewhat painful to let your baby cry for even a minute. If your baby continues to cry for about three minutes while you are gently patting them or rubbing their back, you should pick them up and comfort them by singing to them or talking to them for a few minutes, and then try again to put them down. This routine can try your patience, but if you are consistent with it your baby will learn that when you put him/her in their sleeping place, you are still there and available to comfort them or meet whatever need arises. They will find comfort and security in this and start sleeping without crying.

If at all possible, do not change the bed time or the routine until it is solidly established. Once the bedtime and routine is established, you can occasionally change it when it is absolutely necessary to do so. Sticking to the routine may require some discipline on your part. It will require you to drop whatever you are doing and go through the bedtime routine with your baby. This may mean staying at home in the late evenings, when you'd rather go out. It may mean missing your favorite TV program or leaving office work until the next day. But in the long run it will afford you the freedom to have time for yourself after the baby is asleep. It will also afford you the gift of getting to bed on time each night without your baby fussing. Having a set bedtime allows you to also schedule nights out for yourself with the security of knowing the babysitter can handle getting the baby to bed without any problems.

When your baby wakes up to eat during the night, it is best to leave the lights off and quietly feed and change the baby and get them right back to sleep. In the same way that you established a bedtime routine, establish a night time feeding routine. If you turn on lights and play with your baby during night feedings, they will come to expect this, and even when you are very tired the baby might not go back to sleep for several hours. If your baby establishes this night time play routine, you will quickly become sleep deprived if you have to get up in the mornings.

You can also adopt a nap time routine for getting your baby to sleep during certain times during the day. This will help your baby establish good sleeping patterns and ensure they are well rested without having naps too close to bed time. Established daytime nap routines will help you to schedule your day around baby's naps.

Do not expect your baby to instantly fall into the sleeping routine. It will take some time. Each baby is different, and some babies will take longer than others to fall into a routine, but if you are consistent with the routine, you should notice that your baby is adopting the routine within a week to ten days. Being well rested and having a well rested, happy baby is a wonderful reward for your patience, consistency, and endurance during the time of establishing a routine!

Where and How Should your Newborn Sleep?

Babies should sleep on their back. For many years new parents were told that they should put their newborn face down in the crib or bassinet. But since the "Back to Sleep" campaign in 1994, pediatricians have advised parents to let infants sleep on their backs, both at night and during naps. While new parents worry that the baby may choke on spit-up while on their back, according to a December 2009 National Institutes of Health news release, there is no danger of that. Marian Willinger, PhD, Special Assistant for SIDS research at the Eunice Kennedy Shriver National Institute of Child Health and Human Development, stated, "Placing infants on their backs for sleep remains the single most effective means we know to reduce the risk of sudden infant death syndrome. For the vast majority of infants, concerns about choking while back sleeping are unfounded."

One of the things that new parents may worry most about is Sudden Infant Death Syndrome or SIDS. SIDS is a term that is used to describe the sudden and unexplained death of a baby that is under one year of age. In past times, SIDS was known as Crib Death. No one knows what causes SIDS, but SIDS has been related to certain factors. It is known that babies are more likely to die from SIDS if they are placed on their stomachs to sleep on soft bedding and are covered with heavy or multiple blankets. Most SIDS deaths occur when the baby is less than six months old.

SIDS is not something that you should feel anxiety about, but you should know the risk factors and do what you can to lower the risks. Here are some tips from the American Academy of Pediatricians on how to reduce the risk of SIDS:

✓ Do not smoke during pregnancy or allow your baby to be exposed to second hand smoke after he/she is born, as this can increase risk of SIDS.

✓ Place your baby in a safety-approved crib with a firm mattress and a fitted sheet. Avoid using a soft or lumpy crib mattress.

✓ Never let your baby sleep on a soft surface such as a chair, sofa, water bed, or cushion.

✓ Dress your baby in weather appropriate sleepers that will keep him or her comfortable, and keep the room at a comfortable temperature and avoid using blankets. If you feel you must use blankets while your baby is sleeping, tuck the blanket into the sides of the crib and make sure they do not come up any higher than the baby's chest.

✓ Do not let your baby get too warm while sleeping.

✓ Do not use heavy blankets, quilts, comforters or stuffed toys in the crib.

✓ It is best not to use bumper pads, but if you do, they should be firm and thin and secured to the crib. They should not be puffy pillow-like pads that your baby could press their face against or get their head under to cover their face.

✓ The safest place for your baby to sleep is in their crib or bassinet that is in the room where you sleep, but not in your bed.

✓ Make sure anyone who cares for your baby knows the tips for helping to avoid SIDS.

Feeding Your Baby

Breastfeeding

Before your baby is born, you will need to make a decision about whether you will breastfeed or bottle feed your baby. You may want to talk to your doctor or a lactation specialist about the advantages and disadvantages of breastfeeding. If you are interested in breastfeeding, La Leche League (http://www.llli.org/) is an excellent resource for breastfeeding information. There may also be a local La Leche group with which you can connect.

The American Academy of Pediatrics, among other medical professionals, believes that breastfeeding is the best choice for babies. The AAP recommends that babies are exclusively breastfed for the first six months, and then breastfeeding is continued along with solid foods for the first year (and longer if you decide to breastfeed longer).

Breastfeeding has many advantages:

> ➤ Breast milk is most suited for your baby's digestive system.
> ➤ Breast milk contains all the vitamins, minerals and nutrients that a newborn needs for a healthy beginning and to thrive.
> ➤ Breast milk also contains antibodies that protect your baby from disease and infections during the first several months of their life. Formulas cannot provide these antibodies.
> ➤ Breast milk has long term benefits for baby, including possibly reducing risk of diabetes, asthma, and allergies, and other medical problems.
> ➤ Breastfeeding times are excellent bonding times for mommy and baby.
> ➤ Breastfeeding helps mom burn calories and lose extra weight gained during pregnancy.
> ➤ Breast milk is convenient and instant. There is no need to mix formula, sterilize bottles, shop for formula, and pack around bottles when you go out.
> ➤ Breastfeeding does not affect the family budget in the way that formula does.
> ➤ It is very comforting for mom to know that no matter where she is at with her baby, the milk supply is also there.
> ➤ There is no lugging around a diaper bag filled with formula bottles and risking the formula staying unrefrigerated for too long.

Breastfeeding does require that mom is available and committed to feeding baby. This may mean that sacrifices must be made concerning schedule, job or career, and social life. Breastfeeding moms can get some help with feedings if they pump milk from the breasts with a breast pump and store the breast milk in bottles for someone else to bottle feed the baby. Working moms may express milk for bottles, as well as go home at break and lunch times to nurse their baby. Many women feel the sacrifice they make to get their babies off to a healthy start is well founded.

If you decide to breastfeed your baby, consider purchasing a breast pump so you can pump milk. You may not want or need to do this very often, but it is nice to know that you have an option if you occasionally need one. You will also need to purchase nursing bras and nursing pads. You can purchase washable cloth pads or disposable paper pads to wear inside your bra to absorb milk that leaks when your breasts become full between feedings.

Your newborn does not need to drink water or receive any other nutrition or vitamins while receiving breast milk for the first six months of their life. Although the AAP suggests that breastfed infants are given vitamin D.

At first, your newborn will want to nurse about every one to three hours. Some moms feed on demand (whenever the baby wants to nurse) and some moms choose to feed on a set schedule. In either case, newborn babies should not go longer than about four hours without feeding. When you nurse, try nursing your baby for ten to fifteen minutes from each breast. If you are bottle feeding your baby, give the baby about two to four ounces every two to three hours.

Filled breast milk and formula bottles should be stored in the refrigerator and warmed to room temperature before feeding. Bottles should not be warmed in the microwave, as it can create uneven warming where part of the bottle becomes very hot. You can warm baby bottles in hot water or with a baby bottle warmer. You can fill a crock pot with hot water and let it simmer on low throughout the night to quickly warm bottles in also. You should not store bottles (either breast milk or formula) for more than 24 hours. If your baby does not finish a bottle that has been partially consumed, do not save the unfinished breast milk or formula.

Breastfeeding is very natural, but it can take practice for everything to click for you and your baby. The hospital nurses, a lactation specialist, and your pediatrician will help you learn to feed your baby while you are in the hospital if you need help.

You may feel shy about breastfeeding at first, but once you are used to it, it will become like second nature to you. You'll quickly become a pro at it and your baby will reap all the wonderful benefits of breastfeeding.

Formula Bottle Feeding

Some mothers simply choose not to breastfeed their baby for personal reasons. Women who are under extreme stress or have very demanding careers where they must travel may opt not to breastfeed. In some cases women are not able to breastfeed for health reasons. Examples of those who cannot breastfeed their babies include a mother who is on certain types of medication, or has cancer and is taking chemotherapy. Women with inverted nipples may be told that they will not be able to breastfeed, but lactation consultants can often help these women learn to nurse their babies under this condition. In some instances, the newborn may be sick and not able to feed at the breast. In this event, the mother may be able to pump milk and have it fed to the baby by bottle or a feeding tube.

When a baby is not breastfed, the other option is formula in bottles. Upon arrival home from the hospital, it is important to have bottles sterilized and ready to fill, and a stock of formula to ensure that you do not run out at any time. Your baby will drink about two to three ounces of formula every two to four hours.

It is important that you follow the formula mixing instructions if you purchase the powder formula rather than the premixed kind. If you do not follow the instructions, you are risking your baby not getting all of the nutrients, vitamins and minerals needed for proper growth and development. It is safest to use purified bottled water or boil the water first when mixing baby formula. For the cost of a gallon of purified water or the time it takes to boil water, it is best not to take the risk of contaminated water.

It is important to make sure you buy formula that is not outdated. Always check the container for punctures or dents before purchasing. Follow manufacturer's instructions for storing formula. As with all things concerning baby's food, make sure the utensils and container that you use for mixing formula are clean and sterilized. Most pediatricians feel that running mixing pitchers and utensils through the dishwasher is sufficient.

Using glass pitchers and stainless steel stirring utensils can be more sanitary than using plastic.

Pediatricians often recommend that you feed your baby formula that is fortified with iron. Your baby does not need to drink water or take any additional vitamins or supplements when given formula, unless your pediatrician specifically prescribes something.

If you cannot afford to purchase formula for your baby, or if you are nursing and cannot afford food that will help you sustain nursing, you may want to consider the WIC program. WIC (Women, Infants and Children) is a federally funded program to help provide women and their babies with food for health, proper growth and development. Contact your local health department to find out how to apply for WIC in your state.

Burping

After your baby has breastfed or had their bottle, they will need to burp to expel air they swallowed during feeding. If you do not make your baby burp after feeding, he/she can develop gas pain from gas bubbles. This creates considerable discomfort for your little one, and they will let you know that they are uncomfortable by crying. When a baby is suffering from gas discomfort they may draw their legs upward or try to lie in a curled-up position in order to help expel the gas.

You should burp the baby until he/she is at least six months old, and may want to continue as long as the baby is bottle or breast fed. However, as babies get older and more active they are often able to burp on their own, without help.

There are a few ways to burp your baby:

> ➢ Put a burping pad, hand towel, or a folded cloth diaper over your shoulder to protect your clothing, hold baby vertical with their head on your shoulder and gently pat their back until you hear the burp.

> ➤ Sit the baby on your knee with baby's chin resting in your left hand, while also supporting neck with your left hand. Gently pat the baby's back with your right hand.
> ➤ You can put the baby face down on your left forearm with their face resting in the palm of your hand and their legs straddling your arm at the elbow. Gently pat the back with your right hand. This method only works until the baby gets too long or heavy to securely hold on your forearm. It does not work well if the baby is squirmy. This method of burping seems to be a favorite of dads with strong arms.
> ➤ Often babies will burp more than once, so keep patting and give them an opportunity to burp again.

As babies get a little older they may like to be bounced around and played with after nursing, because they will be happy campers after eating—but it is best to give them time for their milk or formula to settle before the active play starts.

When the baby burps, and at other times too, he/she may spit up a small amount of residual milk. This is normal. However, if your baby spits up a large amount or vomits after feeding for a few times in a row, you should consult your doctor. Your baby may be having some digestive problems or may be allergic to the formula you are using.

Umbilical Cord Cleansing and Bathing

When your baby is in the womb, the umbilical cord is the delivery method for baby's nutrients. Once the baby is born, the nurse, doctor, or often times dad, will cut the umbilical cord and the stump of the cord that is left on the baby will be clamped off until it dries up and falls off, usually within about two weeks old.

The umbilical cord stump can be a concern for the new mom. Rest assured that the umbilical cord stump may look icky, but it does not hurt your baby at all. The baby does not feel the stump at all. It is normal for a little dried blood or crust to be around the stump.

You need to keep the stump clean and dry. Make sure the diaper sits below the stump. You can buy newborn disposable diapers with the front cut lower specifically for the umbilical cord. If you use cloth diapers, simply tuck the front in so that the diaper does not touch the cord. Put a white clean t-shirt under baby's sleeper or clothing to help absorb any moisture that might create the right conditions for infection, and to keep clothing from rubbing against the stump.

> Until the cord dries up and falls off, give your newborn sponge baths instead of baths where baby is immersed in water.

Sometimes the stump will get sticky or your baby may soil the diaper in such a way that it gets on the stump. If the stump needs to be cleaned, wash it with natural soap and water and make sure you dry it very well. It is no longer recommended that you use alcohol to clean the stump, as research has shown that the cord may heal and fall off faster without the use of alcohol for cleaning it.

Do not pick at the cord or try to make it fall off. It will fall off at just the time it is supposed to. Watch for signs of infection, although umbilical cord infections are rare. Call your doctor if the umbilical cord continues to bleed or the area around the cord is red and swollen. Call your doctor if pus oozes from the cord or you if you notice a foul-smelling discharge.

Bathing, Diapering and Dressing

Bathing

As stated earlier, until your baby's umbilical cord stump falls off (when the baby is around ten to twelve days old), you should only give him/her sponge baths. In the case of a baby boy, you should also wait until the baby boy heals from the circumcision before giving a bath other than a sponge bath.

Your baby's skin is sensitive and needs to retain its natural oils. Therefore, it is not good to bathe the baby too often. Two or three sponge baths per week is fine as long as you keep the baby's diaper area clean and dry, and wipe around the mouth and neck area to rid skin of any dripped milk. Remember that bacteria forms in moist, enclosed spaces and that can be a problem if milk drips down the chin and onto the neck or behind the ears.

Gather your baby's clean diaper, clothes, and towels and place them within reach in the area where you are sponge-bathing the baby. Put the baby on his back on a towel, or in a baby bath tub. When sponge bathing, leave the diaper on baby until you get to that area to avoid him/her urinating or pooping while un-diapered. Simply wash the baby using a wash cloth that is wet with warm water and gentle baby soap, if you prefer:

- ✓ Gently wash around baby's eyes.
- ✓ Gently wash behind ears and in neck creases where milk drips and collects.
- ✓ Gently wash outer ears with washcloth or cotton swabs dipped in peroxide or oil. Do not stick cotton swabs or anything else into the baby's ear canal, as you could accidentally puncture the eardrum. There may be wax in the ear canal, but do not try to remove it. The wax is a protective coating for the eardrum, and it will fall out on its own.
- ✓ Wash front and back. This may be a good time to gently massage the baby's back and help them relax.
- ✓ Wash arms and hands, including between fingers. It is normal for "lent" to form between baby's fingers and toes.
- ✓ Wash legs and feet, including between toes.
- ✓ Take off diaper and wash diaper area last.

Be sure you thoroughly pat dry each area immediately after washing. This is particularly important for the diaper area, to avoid diaper rash. Drying baby as you go will keep him/her from getting chilled. Keep in mind that baby can get chilled even on a warm day if left wet and there is a breeze.

To wash baby's hair while sponge bathing, diaper the baby and wrap in warm towel or blanket, so they do not get chilled while you are washing their hair. Dip the washcloth in warm water and wring out slightly, leaving some water for the baby's hair. Add a tiny drop of gentle baby wash or shampoo and gently massage for a few seconds. You will feel the baby's soft spot, but it is perfectly fine for the soft spot to get wet. Rinse the wash cloth and gently rinse the baby's scalp with the wet washcloth. Make sure you remove all soap or shampoo from baby's scalp and hair. Pat hair dry with a towel.

Once the baby's umbilical cord stump falls off, you can bathe your baby in a baby bathtub or a clean kitchen or bathroom sink. Baby bath tubs can be safer in the sense that there is no sink faucet to deal with. However, you must be extremely careful about where you place the baby tub. The tub can be placed on a kitchen or bathroom counter, on a sturdy table top, or in the bathroom bathtub. If you put the baby bathtub on a counter top or table, make sure it is secure and away from the edge, and will not slip off or tip over. Putting a towel underneath the baby tub may help with this.

Get into the habit of following a routine with your baby's bath. This will help you stay organized and focus on a safe and fun bath with baby.

 No matter what happens during baby's bath, never leave the baby in the tub unattended. This means not even for one second! If the phone rings and is not within your reach, simply do not answer it, or take the baby out of the tub and take her/him with you to answer the phone. If there is an emergency, let your first thought be to grab your baby from the tub; no matter what else is going on. Babies can drown in very small amounts of water. Even if an infant is not rolling over, they can turn their head and face into the shallow water and inhale water.

1. Put baby's bathtub in place and make sure it is secure and won't slip or tip.
2. Gather all of the bathing supplies and baby's towel and place next to tub, within reach.
3. Fill the tub with about two to three inches of warm water. (You should not have your hot water heater turned up any higher than 120 degrees to avoid overly hot water that could burn baby if he/she accidentally came into contact with it.) Never leave the water running while you put your baby in the tub. If the temperature of the water suddenly changed to hotter or colder it could scare or hurt your baby.

4. Wash baby all over as described above in sponge bath section on previous page.
5. Pat baby dry with towel.
6. Diaper and dress baby.

Cradle Cap

During the first few months, your baby may develop crusty, flaky patches over their scalp, and sometimes on their eyebrows. This is commonly known as cradle cap, even though the correct name for it is "infantile seborrhea dermatitis". Cradle cap is a normal condition that eventually goes away on its own. Cradle cap does not hurt your baby, nor does it mean that you are not keeping your baby clean enough. If cradle cap appears, you can gently brush your baby's scalp with a baby brush with soft bristles or a baby comb. Do not pick at the crust and try to peel or scrape it off. Anytime you are brushing your baby's hair, remember that there are soft spots.

So what about all of those sweet smelling baby soaps, shampoos, washes, powders, and lotions? Babies do not really need anything more than water for their bath. In fact, some pediatricians warn against using products that may clog pores. If you really want to use lotions to give baby that baby-fresh smell, use very mild baby products—not adult products, and use sparingly, not daily.

Diapering

Whether you are using cloth diapers or disposable diapers, organizing a diapering station can contribute to easy, fast diapering of your newborn. If getting organized to change diapers sounds like overkill to you, you'll probably change your mind after changing dozens of diapers in a week! Everything that you can do to streamline the process is helpful and saves time. You will spend a lot of time changing diapers over the next several months.

You can set up a diapering station in the nursery. Or, you can also set up mini-diapering stations in other areas where you spend time. Toss a small container of disposable diapering wipes or wash cloths, a few diapers, a changing pad and trial sizes of whatever other supplies you need into a medium size basket with a handle, and keep it wherever you are at with baby. This can be particularly helpful when you first come home from the hospital and if you live in a two-story house and you have to go up or down stairs to the nursery.

 Sanitation and safety are the main issues when it comes to diapering. Make sure you do not leave your baby unattended on a changing table or other surface where the baby can roll off. Even if you use the straps on the changing table, do not leave the baby unattended.

Make sure the changing pad is wiped down with a sanitizer after each diaper change or if you use a receiving blanket for changing baby on, toss it in the laundry after each use. Dirty changing mats can grow bacteria that can make you and your baby sick. Make sure you wash your hands thoroughly after each diaper change. It is a good habit to wipe the baby's hands after every diaper change. Particularly, as they get older they will move their arms around and may come into contact with the urine or poop. When changing the baby, double check to make sure poop has not gotten on any of the baby's clothing or on their skin. Babies love to kick when the diaper is taken off and can sometimes get poop on the heels of their feet or socks when kicking.

Check your baby's diaper often and change the diaper as soon as it is wet or soiled. Diaper rash can mostly be avoided if careful diapering is adhered to. It may sound old fashioned, but letting your baby go without their diaper for a few minutes a couple of times each day to thoroughly air out, is an excellent natural deterrent for diaper rash. (If the baby can be in the sunshine and fresh air for a few minutes while un-diapered, it is even better.) If your baby does develop a diaper rash, try using a protective ointment that contains vitamins A and D or apply a protective film of petroleum jelly on their clean, dry, diaper area. If you purchase baby wipes, buy ones without perfumes and dyes. The solution on baby wipes can be somewhat harsh for newborn skin. You can make your own diaper wipes by putting baby oil and a roll of soft tissue paper in a gallon plastic zipper bag so that the tissue paper absorbs the oil.

If you are using cloth diapers, consider the detergent you are washing the diapers in and also let the diapers go through two rinse cycles in the washer to make sure there is no residual detergent left in the diaper. If the diaper rash continues for several days or continues to get worse after you have taken these precautions, talk to your pediatrician about it.

Diapering is fairly simply, though it may be a bit awkward for you the first few times you do it. You'll get plenty of practice, so no worries! Here are simple steps to follow when diapering your baby:

1. Before you unpin or undo the tabs on the soiled diaper, make sure you have everything you need to change your baby's diaper. If you are using cloth diapers, make sure it is correctly folded before you start the changing process.

2. Put your baby on their back on a flat, clean changing surface. Use changing table straps if they are available. You may be tempted to skip the straps when the baby is newborn, but get into the habit of it. It won't be long before your newborn will be squirmy and rolling around.

3. Unpin cloth diapers or undo tabs on the disposable diaper. If you use pins, make sure you put the pins where you can reach them to pin the clean diaper, but where the baby cannot grab them. Always have an extra set of pins nearby.

4. Gently grab the baby's ankles and lift up their legs and bottom. Slide out the soiled diaper and loosely "roll" it up. Put it out of baby's reach until you can properly dispose it off or clean it out for laundering.

5. While you still have baby's legs and behind lifted, use a baby wipe, wet wash cloth or wet cotton pad to thoroughly clean baby's bottom and genital area. You should thoroughly clean baby even if they just wet their diaper. If your baby has been circumcised, follow your doctor's recommendations for cleaning. While cleaning, be careful not to get the umbilical cord stump wet. It is a good idea to gently dry the diaper area after you wipe it. Moisture can create bacterial growth and rashes. As your baby gets fatter, moisture can congregate in folds of skin. Put used wipes or cloths out of baby's reach.

6. Slide the clean diaper underneath baby's bottom. This is a good time to allow baby to "air out" for a couple of minutes to help

avoid diaper rash, especially if you do not dry the diaper area after washing. You can fan the diaper area to help make sure baby is completely dry.

7. Apply diaper cream or ointment on baby if you use it. However, if you change your baby's diapers frequently and make sure they are clean and dry before putting on a clean diaper, as well as let the diaper area air out, rashes will be seldom or nonexistent. The American Academy of Pediatrics recommends you to not use baby powder. It is dangerous for babies to inhale talc powder. Some parents use talc-free cornstarch-based powder as an alternative because cornstarch particles are larger and not as easy for baby to breathe in. But moist cornstarch can help bacteria form. If cornstarch is used, it should be used with caution, and sprinkled into your hand before putting onto baby's skin instead of sprinkling it directly onto baby's skin where it goes into the air and is breathed in by baby.

8. Carefully pin the cloth diaper, or close the tabs of a disposable diaper. If you use cloth diapers, you may be worried about sticking your baby with the pins. Make sure you keep the diaper pins sharp. You are more likely to stick your baby with a dull pin that does not easily glide through the diaper. You can store diaper pins in a bar of soap to keep them sharp.

9. Wash baby's hands and check to make sure there is no poop anywhere on baby's skin or clothing.

10. After removing baby from changing table and putting them down in a safe place, dispose off or clean out soiled diaper and wipes, and thoroughly wash your hands and sanitize changing mat.

If your baby boy has been circumcised, it will take about seven to ten days for the penis to heal afterward. Be sure to gently cleanse the area with plain water every day and during each diaper change. If there is a bandage on the penis, change the bandage each time you change the diaper. Sometimes doctors use a Plastibell to protect the penis instead of a bandage. In this case, the Plastibell should fall off within ten to twelve days. If it does not, you should call your doctor and ask for advice.

You will probably notice a clear crust that forms over the circumcised area. This is normal. A very small amount of blood is also normal on the diaper.

However, if the spot of blood on your baby boy's diaper is bigger than about the size of a quarter, call your doctor immediately. Infections are not common with circumcisions, but watch for any signs such as redness, swelling, yellowish discharge or fever of 100.4 degrees.

Baby's Clothes

Shopping for your baby can be a lot of fun and friends and relatives will want to get in on the fun as well. But keep in mind that your baby will be growing at a rapid rate and each size of clothing will only fit for mere weeks before the baby moves on to the next bigger size. For all practical purposes, a baby does not "need" very many clothes of one size. When shopping, it is fun to look at the frilly girly outfits and the "little man" outfits for your baby. It is fun to "dress up" your baby and show him/her off. Who can resist a baby—let alone one that's all dressed up! But stop and think about how you feel when you are all dressed up for a wedding or formal event. You are probably not very comfortable. You wouldn't want to wear dress-up clothes every day and you certainly wouldn't want to sleep in them. Newborns need clothes that are comfortable and nonbinding and suitable for their many daytime naps. Babies do not usually enjoy getting dressed. Dress-up outfits often have accessories that add to dressing time. So, dress up your baby for special events or for photos, but in general, let their comfort be the rule for choosing what they will wear.

It is best to avoid clothes that have metal zippers and other trims that could scratch or injure your baby. All baby sleepers should be of flame-resistant material. Also avoid putting really baggy clothes that could catch on other things while you are holding your baby. On the other hand, baby's clothes should not fit too tightly or they will be uncomfortable.

Your baby should wear weather appropriate clothing. Natural or natural blend fabrics, such as cotton knits, allow for air circulation and keep the baby at a comfortable temperature in summer months. In winter months, layered breathable clothing that covers your baby's arms, legs, and feet is a good choice. Make sure your baby does not become too warm in blanket sleepers, and remember that some synthetic fabrics do not allow air to circulate and cool your baby if they become too warm.

Babies do not need shoes until they start walking. In the winter socks, booties, or sleepers with feet in them can keep baby's feet warm. Newborns may need to wear light cotton mitts over their hands to help keep them from scratching their face and eyes when their hands flail around uncontrollably.

Change your baby's clothes as needed when they spit up on them or otherwise dirty them, or change them daily. Putting a drool bib on the baby as soon as you change their clothes will help the neck/chest area and front of clothes stay dry when baby drools. Drool bibs are particularly beneficial when baby starts teething and drools non-stop.

What Do I Do When Baby Cries?

New moms may become flustered and worried when their newborn babies cry. It helps if you remember that crying and limited body movements are the only ways that newborns have to communicate with you. They usually cry to let you know that they need or want something. Sometimes babies cry simply because they are tired. They may become fussy because they are over stimulated and the fussiness turns to crying because the baby feels out of sorts and does not know how to communicate. Unless the baby continues to cry for a longer period of time or cries often for seemingly no reason, you can assume that he/she is simply crying to communicate with you, and there is no reason to be alarmed or frustrated.

When your baby cries go down this check list to determine why he/she may be crying:

- ✓ Make sure your baby was not startled or is not hurt. Check for scratches, as sometimes babies accidentally scratch themselves. If you use cloth diapers, check for diaper pins that may have come undone—even though diaper pins have safety covers that help prevent them from coming undone.
- ✓ Check the diaper. Some babies do not seem to mind a wet or soiled diaper so much, but others are easily agitated by it.
- ✓ Check baby's clothes to see if she/he has spit up or if the neck/collar area of their clothes is wet from drool, it may be agitating them.

✓ See if baby is hungry, either by noting the last time she/he was fed or offering the breast or bottle. Nursing babies will often turn their head toward your chest when they are hungry. They may make a sucking motion with their mouth or want to chew on your finger or their fingers when they are hungry.

✓ Try to burp baby. If they are crying and trying to bring their legs up toward their chest or curl up, they may have gas pain.

✓ Hold and cuddle baby close to you to comfort him/her.

✓ Offer a pacifier for baby to suck.

✓ Distract the baby with a toy rattle or by making funny sounds, or by going into a different room or turning on music.

✓ Change baby's position—roll them over on their tummy or sit them up (while you support them of course).

6

KEEPING YOUR NEWBORN
HEALTHY

Soft Spots on Baby's Head

When your baby is born, not all of the bones of the skull will be connected. This is so your baby's head can continue to rapidly grow during the first 18 months of his /her life. (Most of the baby's head growth will occur during baby's first year!) The bones will eventually fuse, but in the mean time, your baby has "soft spots" (fontanel). There are two main soft spots—one is on the back part of the top of the head. This, known as the posterior fontanel, will be completely closed by about four months. The larger anterior fontanel is on the top of the head toward the front of the head. This soft spot usually closes between 12 to 18 months.

Baby's soft spots require no treatment or special care, other than the way you will naturally guard any injury to your baby's head by making sure they do not fall on their head or hit their head on anything or with anything.

Bowel Movements

Talking about bowel movements is not the most pleasant topic—but you will learn that you can tell a lot about your baby's health by his/her bowel movements. You will learn to pay attention to the changes in bowel movements as an indicator of what is going on with your baby's body. In time, you will figure out what is "normal" for your baby and when you should take note. After your baby settles into his/her routine, in the event that your baby's bowel movements suddenly change to very watery or very hard, pay attention and monitor the situation. Call the pediatrician if you do not see any improvement.

Your baby's first stools will be blackish-greenish tarry stools (called merconium). These will last for a day or so, and then you will see loose greenish stools. After that, around day three to five, the baby will have soft stools which are brownish mustard colored. If you are breast feeding your baby, the stools may be loose, and can tend toward a greener color. Your baby will poop their diaper after each feeding for the first several weeks, but will eventually poop only about one to three times per day.

Nasal Passages

Your newborn baby may sneeze fairly often. They sneeze to try to keep their nasal passages clear. Of course babies cannot blow their nose with a tissue like adults do. If your baby's nose is stuffy, it is important to use a nasal aspirator to remove the mucous from baby's nose. You were probably given an aspirator at the hospital when your baby was delivered. If not, they can be purchased at any drug store.

To use the aspirator, squeeze the bulb and continue to squeeze while you gently insert the pointed end into one of the baby's nostrils. Do not push up too far—only the tip needs to go into the nostril. Slowly release the bulb. The aspirator will suck the mucus out of baby's nose. Wipe off end of aspirator and then repeat the process with the nostril. A cool mist vaporizer can also help if your baby develops congestion

Skin

Babies are often born with red marks on their upper eyelids, back of neck and other areas of their body. The marks are harmless and will usually fade over time. Your baby may also develop milia, or tiny white pimples, on their face. Do not pick at or "pop" the pimples as this can lead to bruising and possibly infection. The pimples will disappear within a few weeks. The only skin care your baby really needs is to be gently cleaned with water.

Lowering Risk of Disease and Illness

When your baby comes home from the hospital and when you take him/ her out in public, people will stop and talk to him/ her. People just cannot resist babies. Some will want to touch your baby, and friends and relatives will want to hold your baby and may even kiss the baby on the cheek or forehead. This can be problematic because your baby is being exposed to a lot of germs when he/she is passed around. Babies do build up some natural immunity, but it can be foolish to expose them to whatever sickness others may have. Decide what boundaries you want to set up regarding strangers and others touching or holding your baby, and kindly, but firmly initiate the boundaries. If you do not want family members and friends to kiss your baby, let them know that it's nothing personal, but you have a no-kiss policy in order to keep baby well.

Enjoy Being a Mom!

Nothing can compare to being a mom. You'll experience joy like you never thought possible, and your work and diligence will be rewarded with cute smiles and warm cuddles. Every day won't be all sunshine and fun, but the days that are will far outnumber the challenging days. Enjoy your baby!

DEDICATION

This book is dedicated to my daughter-in-law, Melanie. May the advice in this book give you the confidence to be the best mother you can be.

And to my granddaughter Armella, whose being inspired this book. Without you, life would not be the same.

To my husband, Joseph, for all his love and support through the years.

To all my children who have inspired me and given me the gift of motherhood.

To Jean and Marie-Virginie Kouamou and Marie Patipa for all your wisdom and support.

Author's Bio

Anne Marceline Yepmo, born in Bafoussam, Cameroon, relocated to the United States in 2006. She was the only girl born into a family of five children; she is also the mother of ten. She currently resides in Maryland, where she enjoys spending time with family, especially her granddaughter.